JUICING FOR YOUR SOUL:
An Invitation to Health and Longevity

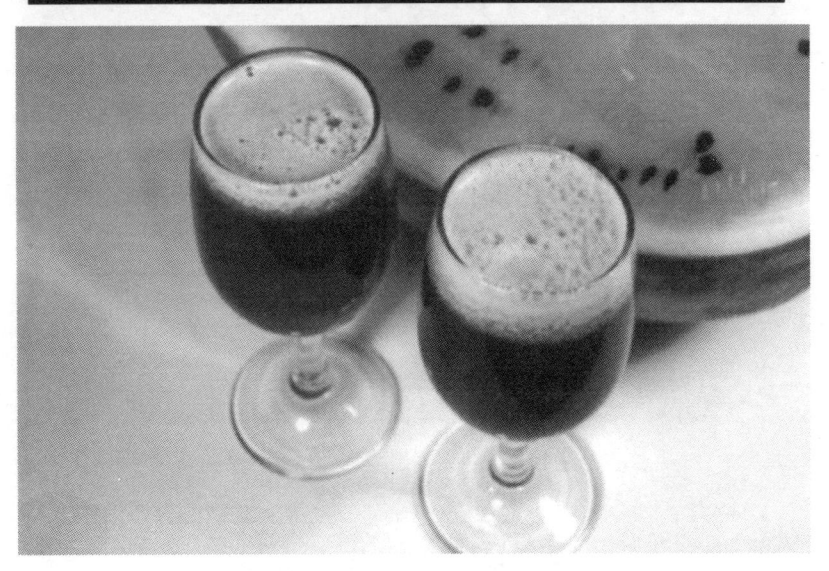

Juiced watermelon rinds

Dedicated to
MY MOTHER
MY FATHER
MY SIBLINGS
AND TO THE LOVELY MAN IN MY LIFE, Dr Jelden

Copyright ©1998-2004 by Phiner Dike.
Published by Phiner Dike
Library of Congress Cataloging-in-Publication Data.
ISBN 0-9643652-6-X

All rights reserved. No part of this publication may be reproduced, stored in a retrieval system, or transmitted in any form or by any means–electronic, mechanical, photocopy, recording, or any other–without the prior written permission of the publisher.

"You pay for your health now or the lack of it later"

Juicing For You Soul

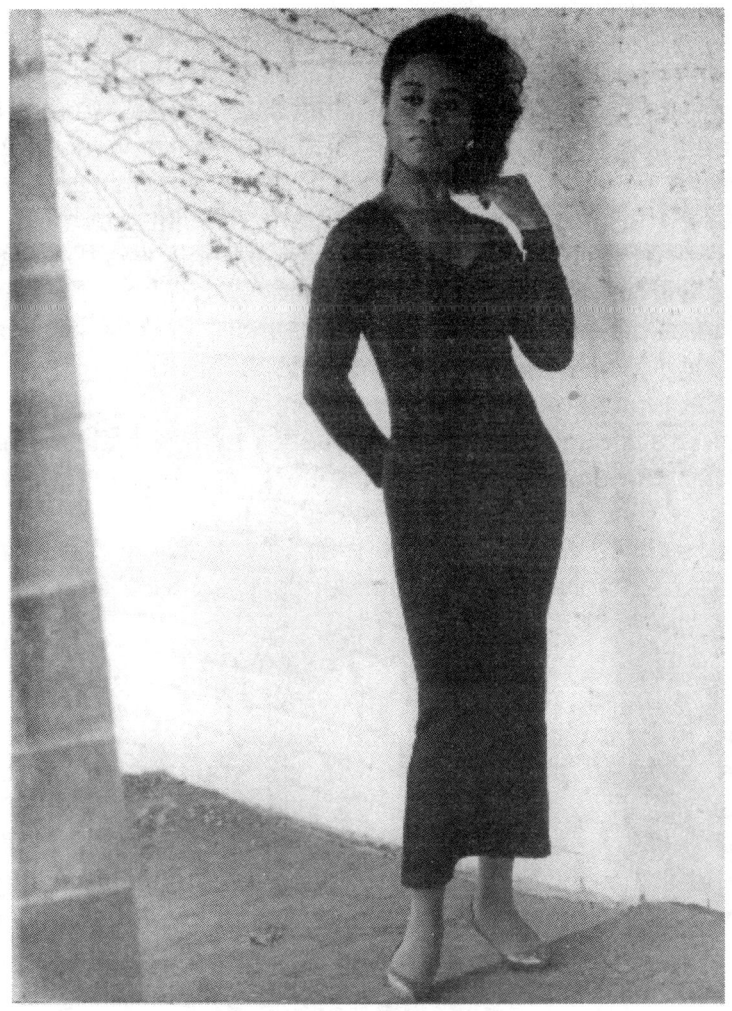

Phiner Dike standing tall

ACKNOWLEDGMENTS

Hi God, it's me, Phiner. Just a note to say: thanks for everything. I am extremely fortunate to know so many people who have been constant sources of inspiration, ideas, and information. It is, therefore, difficult to even know where to begin with these acknowledgments. It is difficult to love with arms open wide enough to hold without crushing, mind clear enough to understand without judging, heart big enough to give without expecting to take. But, that is what my father and mother have done throughout my life. Without their gracious love and support, let alone my modeling and acting career, I would not have had the sense of security and balance that has guided me when my path wasn't clear. It does not seem enough merely to acknowledge my parent's involvement and influence. Yet, all I can say is, they are my light.

Thank you for teaching us how to eat well, how to share, and most importantly, for teaching us that we have to deal with people above us and below in the same manner. We have to show respect. Thank you greatly for our upbringing.

"My heart is oppressed when I see the sin of the world & the whole range of menaces gathering like a dark cloud over mankind. But despite the clouds, my heart also rejoices with hope. We must all do our part to bring peace into the world and into every individual heart.

I would like to thank my wonderful, precious, and lovely siblings, Cosmas, Franco, Oke, Pius, Selin, and Joy Dike for their advice, love, and generosity. You're the nicest, well-mannered siblings anyone could have dreamed to have. I deeply appreciate your honor and integrity you have shown me, you're the pride of my life. I will forever love you all.

Juicing For Your Soul

And then there's Dr. Gwynn Jelden, the love of my life, a truly sophisticated, giving, and caring man. My darling, you're truly a class act. My affections are unalterably yours. I know of no man who would be more acceptable to my parents. Your charming personality is backed up by intelligence and that's so valuable to me. You're the honorable, noble man to whom I will always give my affections. Thank you for all the joys and the encouragement you have given me. Your quiet professionalism has always been a rock of support. You're an epitome of style, grace, and class.

Special thanks go to Charles Walker, whose efforts have added so much to this book. I can't thank you enough for your enthusiasm and ideas.

I am grateful to all my friends around the world for being so nice and always keeping in touch. I am also eternally grateful to Anthonia Okwudibonye, Helen Omogbale, Moji Alajo, Seye Aina, and Toyin Ibiam. Thank you for being the best friends since elementary school. You're simply a class act. Your friendship is invaluable and I will always cherish it for the rest of my life. Thanks for a lifetime of friendship.

Thanks also go to Michell Foster at Cenex Casting in Burbank. Thank you for giving me my first movie opportunity with James Earl Jones and Billy Dee Williams. I had such a wonderful time. Your good spirit will always live in me. I will forever be grateful to you and all the staff I met at Cenex Casting. What a class act you are.

To Carol Mosic, Cindy, and all the staff at Cam Talent agency for giving me my first television commercial opportunity.

To Mr. and Mrs. Joseph Smith for your patience, understanding, love, and confidence in me.

To Najee for your musical support.

I particularly want to thank my friends for being there for me: Rev. Tom Chapman, for your Godly support; Wanetta and family; Attorney Ken Sollarce, for being honest; Larry Vaughn; Commissioner and Mrs. Virgil Brown for your help at the right time.

To all my college professors: you are the best in all intellectual capacities.

To the following people... I always have appreciated and will always remember all that you have done for me. The best way I know to say, "thanks for all you have given me" is to pass it on. For it is in your good names and your memory that I will strive to give something back and pass it on to those who will follow us. I want you to know that you have touched my soul in a way that will be treasured for life. For God's sake–let us continue to work together to win the Human Race.

Brenda Thomas, for adding that special touch and caring.

Bookseller's Staff–Richard Gildenmeister; Howard and Heath Holbert; Peter Cass; Marcelle Nance; Bryce Eiman. Here's to new beginnings.

For the kind words, support, and inspiration: Cindy Hill; Kimyette Finley; Yvonne Gay; Robert Deitchman; Russell Hubbard; Yvonne Marion Cannon; Bill Cherry; Lee Kareem and Family; Jerry Gillett; Marcia Levine, Esq.; Leo Koury; Michael Ross, Esq.; Christine Claussen; Brian McIntyre; Eddie Omobien; Dr. Herbert Kabrin; Larry Calvin; Larry Walters; Kevin Jones; Lucky Upton; Alex Bognoi; John Stuerh; Jonathan Wilhelm; Horst Pfeifer; Judith C. Allen; Toni Driscoll; Nancy Prosser; Florence Hughes; Jean Smith; Ollie Wilson; Brenda Johnson; Torlice Sherrill; Eril Pinson; Theresa Boyd; Theresa Moore; Margaret Saadi; Larry Wallance; Paul Anderson; Peter Grear, Esq.; Marlene and Michael Robinson; Joyce Grear; Chris Tall; Funmi Olinda; Jack Christopher, for always being there; Elizabeth Okwudi;

Juicing For Your Soul

Kalam Muttalib, Esq.; Mr. And Mrs. Juan Wilborne; Ever Jean Stoner; Hap Gray; Richard Virgo; Carol Guest; Mary Stoleriski; Michele Rudolph; Lola Hall; Genelle Gatsons; Mary Massey; Donna Stevens; Valerie Ballom; Luzelle Lewis; George Hill; Elizabeth Pratt; Terry Bush; Vanessa Sykes; Betty J. Thomas; Joanne Sidoti; Jewel Kelley; Catherine Lott; Henrietta Courts; Vashti Armstrong; Judy Fox; Lisa Hall; Michael Hollinger; Sheila Burke; Yvonne Oliver; Mamodou' M. Bodj and Family; Dr. Gibbs; Charlene Lynch; Bill Holland; Maria Hardman; Jewette Johnson; Peter Lawson Jones, Attorney; Dr. Raymond Nwadiuk; Charlie Moore; Seyi Ojofeitinu; C. Y. Ofum; C. Y. Ogbu; Ebenezer and Innocent; Tony and Mary Egbe; Mr. & Mrs. Frank Soadwa; Nadyne Tyrner; Bill and Yvonne Kaczmarek; Jackie Walcott; Shirley Tinsley; Irene Clotman; Gwen Fenty; Marilyn Lilly; Bertha Peet; Greg Walker; Beatric Conyer; Gwendolyn Worthy; Kathleen Blake; Maria Gettys; Sandra A. Hill; Marianne Sordi; Quanetta Harris; Jodi Dearth; Kathy Gudel; Richard Greer; Geraldine S. Wartz; Greg Knox; Frances Cylar; Dorothy B. Cooney and Bridget; Freda Davis; Kim Johnson; Lenora Johnson; Michale L. Robinson; Larry Robinson; Paula McG and Artina Graden; Joan Davis; Brian K. Smith; Elaine Galgany; Heather Dana; Mr. Crosby and Joe Parnel for bringing understanding to my new project.

To Jeffrey and Deloris Mazo; Jim Avery; Chris Conces; Fred Griffith; Ernie Rowell, Jim Coleman; Ann Holloway; Lori Brewer; Steve Hibbard; Chris Walter; Olivia Gates; Anthony Willis; Margie Hodge; Naomi Nobles; Joyce Williams; Richard Thomas; Veronica Woods; Cynthia Goodrum; Peg McGan; Robert Brantley; Alfonza Butts; Mimi Burnett; Nathaniel Spotner; Charles Kwesiga and Family.

To my relatives Helen, Boni, Veronica, Patrick, Christin, Beatrice, and May Oloha; Kizzy Long; LeKan

Juicing For Your Soul

Oguntoyiabo; Verle Marjied; Dr. Lonnie Marsh; Justina Dike and Michael Dike—all this is the result of your early nagging.

Dr. Charles Njoku and family, for the encouragement; Luci Diaz, words cannot express my gratitude; To the staff at Forthwrite Literary Agency–Wendy Zhorne and Nick Griffin, for helping me to understand that it's the quality of work that counts; Ken Maddux, for being a shining example of excellence and for the extraordinary unwavering support; Cheryn Smilen, for your brilliance and encouragement; Tom Katvoski, for trying to keep me on the straight and narrow health road; The Repository staff–Kathie Smith and Scott Heckel, for being my news and information lifeline.

Special thanks to Koula C. Niapas, owner of Something Differerent in Cleveland, Ohio; Joe Hines, for your gracious support and inspiration; Jim Fiedler for going the extra mile for me; Elle Peterson, for being a trailblazer in the industry and passing it on to me; Derrick Lewis, for waiting and for always being there.

To the Watermark Restaurant staff, for your confidence in me and helping me to soar; Megan Kavanagh and Partner Book Distributing staff, for your loyalty, vision, and for being my sounding board; John Churchill, for always having the answers and taking the time; James Lee, for your example and your business seal of approval; Frank and Naana, for the guidance; Isaac Achoja, for the love, inspiration, and support; Tim Mitchell, for your enthusiastic support.

To Al Pratt: Thanks for encouraging me to stretch and to grow. Toni Tipton, Richard Peery, Greg Burnett, not enough words can express my gratitude. Wayne Dawson, Jeff Biletnikoff, may Heaven bless you always. Del Donahoo and family, I am eternally grateful for just being you. Janet Stevens, Fred Stevens, thank you a million times. Zealous Artist Agency Staff–Elle Peterson, Cheryn Smilen, for your brilliance and the encouragement. To Bill Silver "B"

Richards, thanks for your encouragement to stretch and grow. To Paul and Paula Kalamaras, what a great couple, thank you for your time and energy. To Jean Mitchell, Cathy Mitchell, and Ruth Persons, thank you for being special. Also to the Adetu and the Boulieris family for your help at the right time. You're simply classy people.

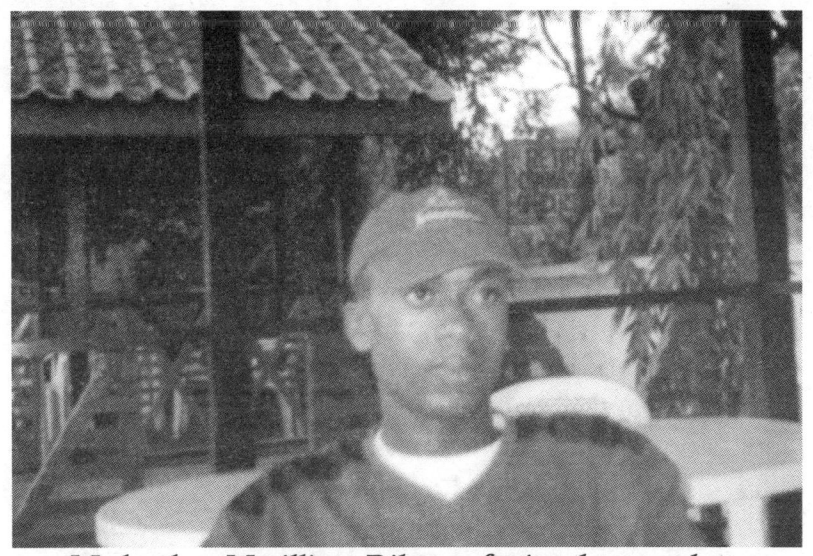

My brother, Macillinus Dike, professional soccer player

FOREWORD
By Charles Cassady, Journalist

Human beings are mostly liquid—at least most of the ones I know are. But how many pay close attention to the liquids that go into our bodies? "You are what you eat," to quote the old saying. What you drink means just as much, if not more, to your physical constitution, mental attitude, and general sense of well-being. Today's market shelves and vending machines are full of dubious, industrial processed brews—our beloved colas among them—that consist of phosphoric acid, alcohol, artificial flavor, artificial color, and artificial goodness. Seriously, read the ingredients label next time you get the chance. It's like a child's chemistry set. Surely that's not what you want to become.

All the more reason to welcome Phiner Dike's *Juicing For Your Soul*, a nutrition manual that explains in plain language and easy recipes how to turn common (or exotic) fruits and vegetables into liquid refreshments that can detoxify and energize the body as well as tantalize the tongue—the wholesome and natural way.

Why not just eat fruits and vegetables as part of your regular meal regimen? Yes, you can do that—but the juicing process means that you absorb the plants' vitamin and mineral benefits in concentrated form. Why contemplate eating a whole grocery cartload of produce when you can get it all in one pitcher? Remember that fruits and vegetables, like you, are largely liquid.

Juicing For Your Soul

    There's an aphorism that "health" is the thing that people are always drinking to—before they fall down. Readers who follow Phiner Dike's advice should not have this problem.

–Charles Cassady
Cleveland, Ohio

INTRODUCTION

The human race has literally enslaved itself. We either robotically or willing commit ourselves and our time to so many activities, most of which have little or no long range value to our overall well-being. If we seek health and fitness we commit to thousands of dollars for equipment, lessons and membership in a golf or country club, or joining a fitness center with perhaps the added cost of a personal trainer. Each such commitment involves driving to and from the place to which you have paid money, so as to put you in touch with what you perceive to be your quest for health and fitness. Just the driving, whatever the distance, is usually aggravating at best, due to traffic, weather or both. If one has young children, they are often plunged into this same self-perpetuating nightmare of 'schedule pressure.' Children are tactfully taught that life is not to be about enjoyment but rather to see how many sports, camps, lessons etc. one can enroll in and parents try to juggle their schedules of work, golf, fitness center, shopping, errands, etc. etc. until it all becomes to overwhelming that one of the first things to suffer is quality family time, or quality personal time if one lives alone. Because most of us think of proper nutrition as too time consuming, healthy eating is something else that usually falls through the cracks. "Drive through, hurry, grab something quick so you can eat before dance class." Very bad lessons for children . . . many of which don't know that this isn't a 'real dinner' . . . or worse yet, not even 'real food'

I know what my body needs because I listen to the signal it gives me. You don't have to go to medical school to nourish and respect your body. If your body is a temple, then you treat it with respect that it is; physical and spiritual.

Juicing For Your Soul

If this book has a bottom line, or theme, it is that you should be living a wonderful life. Whether you're eight years old or eighty years old, you should be feeling alive and invigorated, excited by how wonderful you feel in the world around you. I personally guarantee that this book will meet your highest expectations, because there is nothing like a fresh juice at morning or mid-day as a pick-me-up. Read this book, give it a try, and you'll see that nobody really has a tendency to carry around thirty extra pounds on themselves. And it's not God's fault, either! You are what you eat.

So here in my book, I present ways for you to have ease, convenience, and fun putting a diversity of nutrient-packed drinks into your diet! Hundreds of juicing recipes are included, with an emphasis on fresh fruits and vegetables. Living a good life, where you're vigorous, attractive, and fit, is all about great health. That's what I live by every day, and I'm just as busy as you are.

The constant cry is always, "I don't have time!" We can always make time for what is truly important to us. TAKE some time to assess your priorities. Then arrange them in order of importance. If health is not first, you need to rethink your priorities. Usually the first thing to suffer in this hectic life style we so willingly become bond-slaves to, is the time to get proper nutrition. The excuse for obesity and various illnesses associated with a poor diet is always "I don't have time!" This is the one single reason that fast food has burgeoned into a multi-BILLION-dollar industry. We 'drive thru' the golden arches or another chamber of nutritional horrors, to wolf down some type of mystery meat usually shrouded in breading or tucked into some equally questionable wrap, taco or bun which enables it to be

Juicing For Your Soul

consumed while driving to the next appointment, soccer practice, or Yoga class.

If you will read this book and promise yourself to let its regimen dictate your 'busy schedule' for at least two months, it will be the best gift you could ever give yourself-- the gift of TIME. One can change eating habits in just a few days of working at it, but the secret to making it FAST AND EASY is doing it often enough that it indeed BECOMES your life style. Once you have done this faithfully for six weeks or more you will feel the difference so positively, (and those around you will notice it as well) that its continuation will be self-perpetuating.

Buying the proper fruits and vegetables to prepare and juice as recommended will become so automatic you won't even think of it as 'taking time.' You can make several ounces of healthful, energizing drink in far less time than it takes to get out of traffic and go to the drive thru of some 'Mystery Meat World.' Juicing takes less time than cooking also, and with less clean up. However, properly preparing as a satisfying meal of solid food (yes, as adamant as Phiner is about juicing, for all good reasons, she does also advocate 'chewing'). When you have begun to see and feel the exciting benefits of your primarily juice regimen you will be smiling broadly and far more often. Healthier teeth and gums are just one of the many benefits, so of course when you add to that the enhanced endorphins; the smiles of enjoying your healthy life will keep the smiles coming, so Phiner has other cookbooks which will afford you lots of delicious, healthful chewing.

As you read this wonderful book and reinforce your commitment to yourself, think of the time it takes to change your life style for the greater good, not as a cost of time, but rather as an investment of time, which will bring you the

Juicing For Your Soul

return of health and happiness. You may even decide to skip the golf, tennis, fitness center time and expense, in favor of quality time walking parks or city streets with your children, a loved one, or alone. Time alone is good, and the better you feel and look, the more enjoyable and productive that time to yourself will be. And you won't have to drive anywhere at some appointed time to make it happen.

So, read ***Juicing for Your Soul***, and promise yourself better health, and commit enough time (preferably two months) to adjust your thinking as well as your life style. To know that it is not about 'dieting' and 'counting calories'…even if weight loss is your goal, it will automatically follow when you allow good nutrition to guide you, and if for no other reason than **YOU'RE WORTH IT!**

You can visit my website at www.phinerdike.com or
Reach me by e-mail at phinerd@hotmail.com

Respectfully,
Phiner Dike

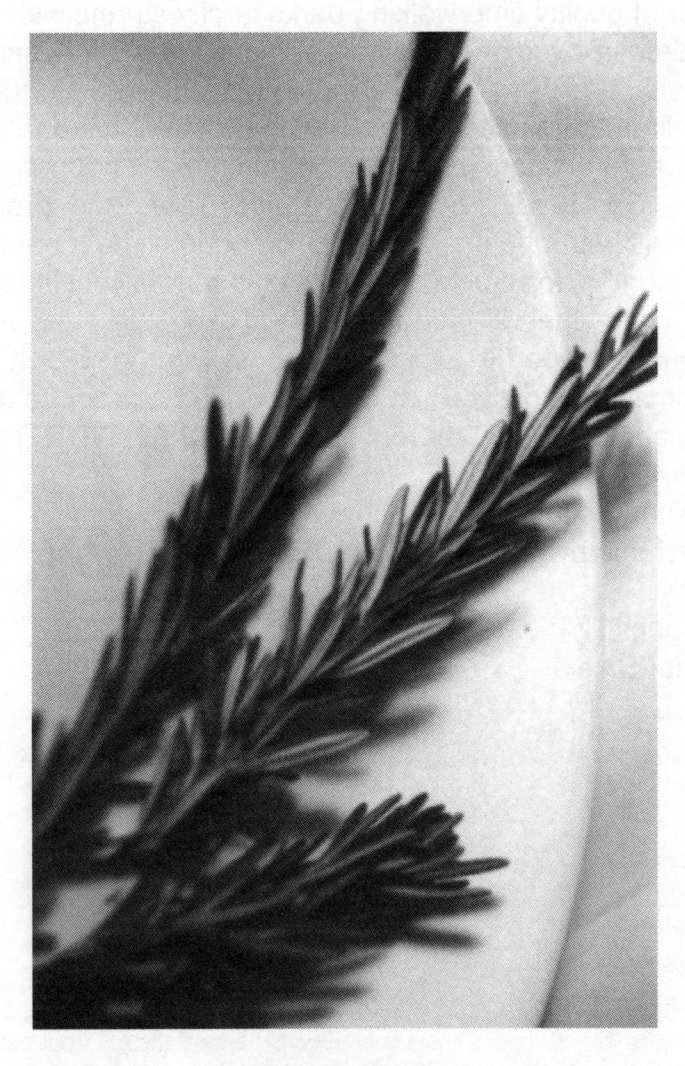

Fresh Rosemary

A Nutrition Summary of the Fruits and Vegetables Used In This Book

Alfalfa Sprouts
Alfalfa sprouts are high in vitamin C, an antioxidant that helps protect the body tissue from chemical stress and is essential for healthy bones, gums and blood vessels. Alfalfa also contains vitamin E, another potent antioxidant that helps stabilize cell membranes and regulates oxidation reactions in the body.

Recipes with alfalfa sprouts can be found on pages 50, 62, 101, 114, 118.

Apples
Apples are full of fiber, which is useful for eliminating all of the toxins in your system. Actually, one twist I've discovered is that when it works, it works—meaning for those who eat three apples a day, the thing is amazing. A healthy colon depends on fiber, which also provides regularity. You can juice all the apples you want, so you should never be hungry—and the pounds fall away.

Recipes with apples can be found on pages 57, 66, 74, 76, 84, 86, 97, 102, 114, 134, 158.

Apricots
Apricots contain silicon, a mineral that gives structure to all living things. Silicon is essential to the human body. It gives strength and support to nails, skin, connective tissue, tendons and ligaments. Apricots could well become the juice to incorporate into your diet if you want health and vitality. Apricots contain an appreciable amount of iron, a vital mineral for strengthening bone, nails, and teeth.

Recipes with apricots can be found on pages 45, 97, 100, and 126.

Asparagus
This vegetable contains a valuable source of potassium, which is necessary for healthy heart rhythm, muscle contractions, and nerves. Asparagus is also a nutritional powerhouse. It is high in folic acid, which prompts the production of red blood cells. For this particular reason, asparagus can prevent and treat anemia due to folic acid deficiency.

Recipes with asparagus can be found on pages 49, 51, 55, 91, and 129.

Basil
Basil is an herb that has some amazing healing properties. It quells nausea and eases motion sickness, among other things. It contains fairly potent anti-inflammatory substances. Basil leaves are effective for treating anxiety and emotional problems.

A recipe with basil can be found on page 60.

Bean Sprouts and String Beans
Bean sprouts and string beans are a rich source of mucilage, a fibrous material that can end the misery of constipation. Not only do bean sprouts enlarge and soften stools and stimulate bowel contractions, but they also help to lubricate their passage. These vegetables enjoy a reputation as a purifier—they increase the flow of urine and promote sweating, all of which rid the body of toxins. In the process, they may also sooth the swelling, inflammation, and pain of arthritis. String beans are excellent for diabetics because they regulate blood sugar

Juicing For Your Soul

and lower cancer rates. They are high in fiber, which makes them important for functions of the colon, hemorrhoids, and other bowel problems. String beans contain vitamin A, a key building block for keeping the urinary lining healthy.

A recipe with bean sprouts/string beans can be found on page 80.

Beets
Beets contain copper, an essential mineral for a healthy immune system, red blood cell formation, hair, and the elastin of muscle fibers. They aid in the conversion of the amino acid tyrosine into a dark pigment (melanin) that colors the hair and skin. Beets also contain calcium, the most prominent and well-known mineral for producing healthy bones and teeth, but it is involved in many other vital processes including heart, nerve, and producing many enzymes. Beets help with muscle cramping, nervousness, and tingling, besides bone structure.

Recipes with beets can be found on pages 48, 70, and 71.

Blackberries
Blackberries contain magnesium, an incredible mineral so wonderful for eliminating muscle cramps, tension and nerves. They also contain vitamin C, an amazingly versatile remedy for virtually everything. Vitamin C can be used for accelerating healing of wounds, fighting viruses, controlling allergies, and detoxifying the body.

Recipes with blackberries can be found on pages 116, 144, 147, and 157.

Blueberries
Blueberries are one of the most remarkable antioxidants because they are involved in the energy production system. They also contain vitamin A, which can reduce sebum production, therefore reducing the likelihood of pimple formation. Blueberries are one of nature's best tranquilizers containing a sedating compound—flavonoids—that also relieve muscle tension and insomnia.

Recipes with blueberries can be found on pages 75, 95, 137, 143, and 148.

Broccoli
Broccoli contains the vitamin B complex that will help keep the fragile system of nerves, nerve sheaths, and synapses healthy and responsive to stimuli. The central nervous system relies heavily on vitamin B_6, part of the B-complex to assist in the production of serotonin, a critical neurotransmitter. The B-complex vitamins will also maintain proper electrical energy and nutrient transfer across cell membranes. Broccoli is loaded with antioxidants. It helps breast, colon, and lung cancer, speeds estrogen removal, and is an anti ulcer remedy as well.

Recipes with broccoli can be found on pages 56 and 84.

Brussels Sprouts
Brussels sprouts are members of the cruciferous family and they fight cancer and regulate hormones. They contain valine, lysine, and methionine, which are amino acids. Valine, an essential amino acid found in muscle tissue, is vital for tissue repair. This particular amino acid can be helpful to drug addicts. Lysine is another essential

amino acid that can be very helpful for children as it may aid in normal growth and development. People who are recovering from either sports injuries or surgery can find this beneficial. Methionine has the ability of breaking down fats, hence, preventing the build up of the fats in the liver. Overweight folks can find this beneficial to them. Really, Brussels sprouts are one of my favorite vegetables.

A recipe with brussels sprouts can be found on page 55.

Burdock Root
Burdock root is an herb that is so useful for providing relief to swelling, inflammation, and pain of arthritis due to its nutritional compound. Burdock root also promotes hair growth and I am living proof.

Recipes with burdock root can be found on pages 88 and 92.

Cabbage
Cabbage is another cruciferous vegetable. People who are trying to shed off some pounds can find it useful, but to receive its full benefits you must, of course, juice it or eat it. Cabbage contains sulfur, a mineral that is crucial to many different body functions and, more importantly, will slow the aging process. With proper exercise and positive mind, cabbage should help you look healthy.

Recipes with cabbage can be found on pages 50, 61, 101.

Cantaloupe
Cantaloupe to me is a wonder cure, but in this case, you must juice everything from the skin, the rind, and the seeds to get the full benefits. It is a powerful antioxidant that will prevent cancer by cleaning the internal cells. It also helps curb hunger. Personally, when I drink

Juicing For Your Soul

cantaloupe juice, I can go for about eight hours without getting hungry!

A recipe with cantaloupe can be found on page 128.

Carrots
Carrots, in general, work by strengthening our immune system. They contain beta-carotene which, when consumed, will convert into vitamin A in our body. The vitamin A will help protect eyesight and strengthen mucous membranes. Carrots are loaded with nutrients. They also cleanse the digestive tract, further helping to rid your system of germs.

Recipes with carrots can be found on pages 47, 52, 62, 69, 75-77, 79, 81, 84, 87, 106-107, 109, 116, 119-120, 122, 130, 145, and 157.

Catnip Leaves
Catnip leaves are useful for people who are suffering from stress, insomnia, joint pain, and indigestion. They contain vitamin B_5, also known as pantothenic acid. One of its major functions is the ability to release energy from carbohydrates and fats. The B_5 vitamin can be helpful in detoxifying alcohol. If you are under heavy stress, you will find catnip leaves useful by incorporating them into your daily diet. Catnip leaves also contain vitamin B_1, necessary for enhancing circulation in our body and it can increase our overall energy level.

A recipe with catnip leaves can be found on page 56.

Celery
Celery is another favorite of mine. Its main function includes, but is not limited to, reducing swollen feet. It is

Juicing For Your Soul

one of the best vegetables to juice for a cigarette smoker as it acts as a detoxifier. It contains sodium which, when consumed, should eliminate the need for consumption of any processed salt. The sodium content of the celery is an important mineral that regulates water balance in the body; hence, you can see why it is important to drink at least a glass of celery juice a day, especially for those whose feet are always swollen. But, again, it is important you move around and avoid sitting for longer than two hours.

Recipes with celery can be found on pages 72, 86, 90, 131, and 146.

Cherries
Cherries are rich in potassium and vitamin C. The mineral potassium can be helpful for people with heart problems and high blood pressure. Potassium can help prevent cancer since it tends to normalize cell growth. The C vitamin can help slow the onset of visible signs of aging, prevent many disorders, and extend life expectancy if you follow my rules of the good life in this book.

A recipe with cherries can be found on page 84.

Chives
Chive is very similar to onion in taste and flavor. Chives have essential nutrients and have stronger disease fighting capability.

Recipes with chives can be found on pages 156 and 159.

Cilantro
Cilantro is useful for appetite stimulation, bad breath, and hemorrhoids. It is also a digestive aid and can lessen

menstrual cramps. It contains vitamin C that aids in forming red blood cells and prevents hemorrhaging. In addition, the vitamin is used in preventing and treating the common cold.

A recipe with cilantro can be found on page 91.

Collard Greens
Collard greens contain vitamin E, which is needed to protect the cells from harmful free radicals. Vitamin E can be of vital importance to people with cardiovascular problems or athletes as it strengthens the heart muscle. Another main contribution of the E vitamin is the healing of scar tissue and it can make a difference on laugh lines. Collard greens also contain vitamin C, an important element that can shield your entire body. It helps make collagen, the glue that strengthens skin, muscles, and blood vessels.

A recipe with collard greens can be found on page 90.

Cranberries
Cranberries are high in vitamin C, which is vitally important for many functions in the body. It is involved in immune system health and collagen formation. Collagen is good for bones, teeth and skin. Vitamin C is also a super antioxidant protector that helps fight cell-damaging free radicals. It helps support the immune system during winter.

Recipes with cranberries can be found on pages 99, 111, 132, and 153.

Juicing For Your Soul

Cucumbers
Cucumbers assist in wound healing. They keep the lining of the nose, throat, lungs, and mucous membranes very healthy. Cucumbers contain beta-carotene that protects the skin from damaging sunlight.

Recipes with cucumbers can be found on pages 63, 65, 78, 85, and 139.

Dill
Dill is an herb, which contains some nutrients that may help the liver filter out toxins more effectively. It also contains manganese, a mineral used for maintenance of healthy sex hormone production and enzyme activation. Dill can greatly relieve sore, itchy eyes due to allergies. It is especially good for those who suffer from hay fever.

A recipe with dill can be found on page 103.

Dandelions
Dandelion leaves are such wonderful herbs packed with energy-giving nutrients. It is an herb I call the energy exchange. It strengthens a host of internal organs, for example, the liver and the pancreas. It will, as a whole, clean the urinary system. It contains vitamin B, known for its role in cellular respiration; thereby keeping the machinery that turns food into energy running. Having trouble staying healthy? Do you feel tired? Are your defenses run down? One thing you must bear in mind if your immunity is weak—you are vulnerable to germs, bacteria, and a host of other diseases that seemingly attack from every angle. Dandelions are rich in natural nutrients to boost all aspects of immunity working together to ensure good health.

Recipes with dandelions can be found on pages 58 and 70.

Endive
Endive is a vegetable loaded with vitamins A, B_5, and folic acid. The vitamin B_5 (a.k.a. pantothenic acid) is a member of the B complex family and is important for resistance to stress, it stimulates growth and the adrenal glands. It may also be useful in treating eczema and diarrhea. The A vitamin is important for treatment of eye and skin problems. No one should fool around with his or her eye problems. Any inflammation, redness, or irritation could be a sign of infection, and that is a potential threat to vision. For minor eyestrain, inflammations, and other ailments, it is worth trying this vegetable first. If it is a major eye problem, see your doctor ASAP. The folic acid provides the gastrointestinal (GI tract) a healthy intestinal flora by keeping harmful bacteria away. Folic acid can help stimulate production of bile salts that defend against harmful invaders and improve digestion of essential immuno-nutrients.

A recipe with endive can be found on page 158.

Garlic
Garlic is in a class by itself due to all its healing natural properties. It is an indispensable feature and should be consumed at least four times a week. It is a healer, capable of treating wounds, aiding digestion, protecting the liver and heart, and easing arthritis pain. Garlic—once again—relaxes the windpipe, which may make it useful for asthma sufferers, as well as other respiratory ailments such as colds and flu. Traditionally, folk healers recommend this herb for coughs and bronchitis. It soothes frayed nerves because it actually slows down the central

nervous system. Garlic contains all the vitamins, minerals, and essential amino acids. Try adding it in any of the juicing remedies when you are feeling uptight. It also has the added benefit of easing the indigestion that may accompany your anxious state. Before going to bed at night, I usually juice four cloves with three oranges, which makes me sleep like a newborn baby.

Recipes with garlic can be found on pages 57, 64-65, 76, 79-80, 88-91, 113-115, 117, 133, 136-139, 143, and 149.

Ginger
Ginger is an herbal root and is a good source of choline and vitamin B_3. Choline is a vitamin that may minimize excessive deposits of fat in the liver. Choline may provide relief for people with thyroid, bleeding stomach ulcers, and nervous problems. Vitamin B_3 can help nervous disorders. It will also provide energy and maintain healthy skin. Ginger roots can help dissolve the type of blood clots responsible for heart attacks and strokes. It also cleanses the colon. It has a powerful antioxidant for cramps, circulatory problems, morning sickness, and nausea.

Recipes with ginger can be found on pages 72, 82, 92, 107, 110, 121, 140, 151, and 158.

Grapes
Grapes contain essential amino acids, the building blocks of proteins that provide structure for all living things. Proteins are important for the growth of bones. The red grapes with seeds are better for you due to the high content of antioxidants. They inhibit blood clotting and raise the good cholesterol. Grapes have the capabilities of stimulating the immune system, the uterus, and the digestive tract.

Recipes with grapes can be found on pages 83, 87, 96, and 147.

Grapefruits
Grapefruits are full of natural nutrients such as vitamin C which can help slow the onset of visible signs of aging. They will help protect the lungs from damage and will act as a block to bacteria and infection. Grapefruits can help reverse clogged arteries, fight stomach cancer, and they lower blood cholesterol.

Recipes with grapefruits can be found on pages 1109, 112, and 143.

Honeydew
Honeydew is high in vitamin A, which promotes healthy cell and tissue reproduction and maintains strong bone and muscle systems. Honeydew juice is so filling and satisfying, thereby making one feel less hungry. It is easy to lose weight with honeydew juice as it also provides more energy than usual. It contains antioxidants that protect the cells from free radical damage, therefore preventing premature aging. It also contains beta-carotene that strengthens the immune system.

A recipe with honeydew can be found on page 55.

Kale
Kale has a beneficial effect on health. Kale has in it rich nutrients that are critical for cell membrane integrity, healthy immune system, maintaining a healthy cholesterol level, and for healthy skin and nails. Kale is a vegetable that is a rich source of vitamin C and is essential for women's issues. It can help to promote healthy hormonal balance, as well as alleviate symptoms from PMS,

Juicing For Your Soul

menopause, hot flashes, and arthritis. It also contains fiber, a support for overall gastrointestinal health.

Recipes with kale can be found on pages 52, 134. and 162 (as a substitute for ugu leaves).

Kiwis
Kiwis store a powerhouse of nutrients that contain potassium and vitamin C, as well as calcium. The C vitamin enhances the brain and eye development and alleviates symptoms of cardiovascular disease, schizophrenia, digestive problems (such as Crohn's), and depression. Calcium is a mineral that will also enhance cardiac muscle and may help prevent bone loss associated with osteoporosis. Potassium, another essential mineral, can help maintain stable blood pressure.

Recipes with kiwis can be found on pages 77, 81, 111, 154, and 157.

Kohlrabi
Kohlrabi is a vegetable that contains all the essentials and has the ability to fire up your body's metabolic rate, so fats move out of your body more efficiently. It also helps to control food cravings and intake, so you can improve your weight. It also contains vitamins A, B_1 and B_2, well known for their powerful antioxidant action–providing the tools to shield and protect you against various diseases and premature aging.

A recipe with kohlrabi can be found on page 151.

Lemons
Lemons have the highest amount of bioflavonoids, which are important for all of the metabolic pathways in the body and all of the chemistry for energy in the body. They are also necessary for building resistance to infection and lowering cholesterol.

Recipes with lemons can be found on pages 58, 66-67, 69, 77, 84, 93, 119, and 140.

Limes
Limes are in the same class as lemons. They contain antioxidants that can block or shrink tumors. They contain some amount of vitamin A that can help support your internal immune system and preserve its valuable balance.

Recipes with limes can be found on pages 58 and 62.

Mangoes
Mangoes are essential to good health, winning the battle for energy and vitality. They contain biotin, B vitamins, and the mineral zinc, which are all essential for healthy hair and skin because of their ability to build protein from amino acids. They are also full of fiber, a remedy for cleansing the colon.

Recipes with mangoes can be found on pages 105, 115, 124, 144, and 148.

Marjoram Leaves
Marjoram leaves are herbs that can help relieve menstrual cramps. They are rich in vitamin A, which can lower the risk of certain eye diseases that result from aging. They

also contain potassium used primarily as a stress reliever and muscle relaxant.

A recipe with marjoram leaves can be found on page 144.

Nectarines
Nectarines contain mega doses of nutrients in phosphorus, magnesium, and other minerals and vitamins. Phosphorous, a remarkable trace mineral is valued for providing energy and vitality. It also provides strength to the bones and teeth. Magnesium is also known to be a component in the development of bones and teeth and may possibly help in their preservation.

Recipes with nectarines can be found on pages 104, 146, and 154.

Onions
All onions, including scallions, chives, shallots, and leeks, are rich in B vitamins and may influence your energy level, mood, and behavior. They may also prevent disorders of the nervous system. Onions are useful for many diseases and illnesses, as they are a potent immune system stimulant and a natural antibiotic. Onions have zero cholesterol, are very low calorie, and have zero fat. They thin blood and inhibit stomach cancer due to their antioxidant properties.

Recipes with onions can be found on pages 52, 93, and 143.

Oranges
Oranges are my all-time favorite. Every night before I go to sleep, I always juice three oranges as they lower blood cholesterol and definitely fight viruses. In combination with

garlic, oranges can be employed to relieve the aches of flu and improve digestion. Folic acid and inositol can be found in oranges, where they perform vital functions in virtually all of the body's systems.

Recipes with oranges can be found on pages 53, 60, 72, 76-77, 80, 94-96, 100, 102, 105, 112, 115-116, and 153.

Papaya (Pawpaw)
Papaya, called pawpaw in Nigeria, is extremely high in vitamins A, C, and the mineral potassium. They contain enzymes that can easily break down protein and starches in the stomach, thereby making digestion easy. Potassium will strengthen your heart and muscles. It will maintain the mineral balance of your blood and a stable blood pressure. The vitamin A will enhance your new cell growth and help fight any infection. It will also help your skin to be healthy and glowing. The C vitamin certainly will help the collagen in your skin and keep it youthful.

Recipes with papaya can be found on pages 46, 67-68.

Parsley
Parsley is an herb, which contains rich nutrients that help regenerate and detoxify your liver. The liver is perhaps the most abused organ in the body. If you consume alcohol or smoke cigarettes, parsley should be part of your daily diet. Parsley is very high in vitamin C, which helps to protect the body against harmful effects of alcohol and pesticides. Parsley also contains essential amino acids that can maintain the health of your liver by making the job of the

Juicing For Your Soul

liver easier. The essential amino acids are also powerful antioxidants by protecting against free radicals produced by alcohol metabolized in the liver.

Recipes with parsley can be found on pages 70, 119, and 151.

Peaches
Peaches contain calcium, a mineral that is necessary to protect your bones, muscles, and joints from deteriorating. As your bone structure deteriorates, it becomes brittle and fragile. Calcium can slow down your bone loss and reduce risk of osteoporosis. You need to bear in mind that your bones change every two years, especially as you get older. Peaches also contain a significant amount of vitamin A, necessary for creating high energy levels and extend youthfulness.

Recipes with peaches can be found on pages 67, 73, 77, and 99.

Peapods
Peapods have amazing healing properties. They may help lower your glucose levels. If you are a diabetic, they are a useful addition to your current treatment plan, but speak with your doctor first. This nutrient-rich vegetable is definitely good for your overall general health. They can certainly help you re-establish regularity.

Pears
Pears are nutritious fruit for improving your bowel movement. They are high in nutrients that provide a powerful fat emulsifier. They also contain vitamin C, which will protect the body from viruses and bacteria. The C vitamin will also maintain clear breathing in the lungs, bronchioles, and the sinuses. Pears also contain

potassium that is essential for your heart. Diabetic people are safe to juice pears, as the sugar is more easily tolerated than other fruits.

Recipes with pears can be found on pages 54, 74, 87, 99-100, 105, 149, and 156.

Peppermint Leaves
Peppermint leaves are nutritious herbs that will soothe and relax your nerves due to their tonic content. They abound in vitamins and minerals that the body needs. They relieve constipation and may generally improve hormonal production in our body. They contain powerful antioxidants such as vitamin C, known to protect our cells by scavenging free radicals, binding to them, and thereby carrying them out of our body!

Recipes with peppermint leaves can be found on pages 59, 76, 85, 98, 102, 107, 110, and 121.

Peppers (green, red, yellow, purple)
Peppers are all highly nutritious and are full of vitamins, minerals, and essential amino acids with zero cholesterol and saturated fats. Peppers also contain a high amount of beta carotene, especially the red ones, an antioxidant that works with other natural protectors to defend our cells from harmful free radical damage caused by highly reactive substances that either form in our body or are acquired from the environment such as air pollution, cigarette smoke, etc. Externally, I have used the pulp as a facial for tightening purposes.

Recipes with peppers can be found on pages 86, 91-92, and 94.

Juicing For Your Soul

Pineapples
Pineapples have so much to offer. Pineapple juiced with the skins on can treat an extensive range of health problems, including pain and inflammation, sinus infection, flu, menstrual problems, constipation, migraine and less severe headaches, heart disease, and skin disorders. They are rich in fiber, which helps cleanse the colon. They also have all the nutrients to slow down the onset of aging.

Recipes with pineapples can be found on pages 46, 74, 125, 135, 137, 141, 148, and 155.

Plums
Plums contain antioxidants such as beta-carotene and vitamin C to help protect the insides of your arteries and veins from disease-producing oxidizing agents. They also contain calcium, a mineral for normalizing blood clotting and essential for rhythmic heart action. Calcium is also vital for strong bones and teeth, as well as for muscle growth.

A recipe with plums can be found on page 81.

Potatoes
Potatoes are relatively high in vitamins B_1 and B_3, as well as iron and potassium. The vitamin B_1 in the potato will provide our body the energy it needs, as well as a healthy nervous system. The B_3, on the other hand, provides us with healthy skin and a healthy digestive system. The mineral iron supplies us with blood quality and increases resistance and energy. Iron can also improve blood circulation. Potassium—this mineral can help strengthen

the heart. It may also prevent cancer growth, as it tends to normalize cell growth.

Recipes with potatoes can be found on pages 65 and 105.

Radishes
Radishes, rich in natural sodium, are used in every cell of our body, thereby helping to regulate our heart, as well as providing balanced fluids. Radishes are a well-respected vegetable and thus lower blood pressure. They are effective in liver cleansing, promoting the secretion of bile due to its rich contents of vitamins, minerals, and essential amino acids.

Recipes with radishes can be found on pages 49, 72, 109, and 120.

Raspberries
Raspberries are one of the most nutritious fruits on the face of the planet Earth. They contain some amounts of niacin, known as vitamin B_3, and some phosphorus. Phosphorus, an important mineral, will repair and maintain the integrity of our cells and provides us with energy. Phosphorus is also vital for skeletal growth and tooth development. Niacin helps to flush out toxins in the body. It can also be used to treat high cholesterol.

Recipes with raspberries can be found on pages 98, 110, 115, 136, and 142.

Rosemary
Rosemary is a nutritious herb with a reputation for enhancing our memory. It is one of the best herbs for treating indigestion, sore throat, muscle and joint pain. It

Juicing For Your Soul

contains some magnesium, a key element for healthy bones, nerves, and muscles.

A recipe with rosemary can be found on page 50.

Sage (Sage Leaves)
Sage, an herbal nutrient, can be used for treating a wide range of gynecological problems. It contains nutrients that can quell painful menstrual cramps, ease or eliminate the symptoms of PMS, soothe hot flashes and other symptoms of menopause. It also has tranquilizing properties which can depress the central nervous system, thereby eliminating stress-related complains or problems.

Recipes with sage can be found on pages 58, 65, 125, and 168.

Scallions (see Onions)

Spinach
Spinach—one of my all-time favorite vegetables. This is a powerhouse of antioxidants such as CoQ_{10}, beta-carotene, and is also extremely high in fiber. It also contains a trace mineral called selenium that will strengthen your muscle tissue and the heart muscle. The fiber in the spinach can help eliminate unwanted toxins in our body and can also lower blood cholesterol. Spinach will help maintain healthy cholesterol levels in our body. The CoQ_{10} produces the basic energy component of the human cell and neutralizes harmful free radicals in our cells. In a nutshell, spinach contains all the rich, key nutrients to fight virtually any aliments from colon cancer to wrinkles.

Recipes with spinach can be found on pages 48, 59, 64, 82, 89, 108, 123, and 130.

Juicing For Your Soul

Strawberries
Strawberries are extremely beneficial to every one of us, but especially if you are a cigarette smoker or work in a polluted environment such as a plant or factory. They contain pectin, a fiber that is important for removing toxins from the bloodstream. Another very useful ability of strawberries is their capacity for fighting cold sores due to their high vitamin C content.

Recipes with strawberries can be found on pages 46, 67, 69, 148, and 150.

String Beans (See Bean Sprouts or Peapods)
Sweet Potatoes (See Yams)

Swiss Chard
Swiss chard is full of vitamin A and the minerals calcium and potassium. The A vitamin is highly essential for the growth of tissue, teeth, and bones. It can also be very beneficial for anyone with vision problems and mucous membrane problems. Another vital function of the A vitamin is the fact that it has anticancer properties. The mineral potassium may benefit those with high blood pressure, heart, and nerve problems. The calcium, on the other hand, can be beneficial to people suffering from osteoporosis by increasing their bone density.

Recipes with Swiss chard can be found on pages 88 and 94.

Tangerines
Tangerines are loaded with essential amino acids. Tangerine juice supplies more vitamin C than oranges. As you may already know, vitamin C is crucial to your overall health, especially to your skin, teeth, gums, muscles, joints, and immune system. One of the essential amino

Juicing For Your Soul

acids in tangerines that I'd like to discuss here is lysine, which contains an anti-aging factor. Lysine may supply the body with blood circulation, high energy, and a strong immune system. Here's to your fountain of youth!!!

Recipes with tangerines can be found on pages 73 (as a substitute for oranges), 83, 99, 111, 133, 136, 139, 144-145, 147, 150, and 156-157.

Tarragon
Tarragon is an herb for stimulating your appetite and relieving indigestion. The rich nutrients in the tarragon can or may help a heart disease patient due to its prevention in the narrowing of the artery wall. It contains a significant amount of the mineral potassium, helping your liver to stay vital and healthy. Another interesting function of potassium is the ability to invigorate and stimulate our liver.

A recipe with tarragon can be found on page 146.

Tomatoes
Tomatoes contain phosphorus and sodium-nourishing elements. For the human heart to function at a normal peak rate, the mineral phosphorus is highly needed. It is also needed for healthy bones and teeth. Tomatoes are rich in nutrients such as antioxidants which can help protect the cells from damage, prevent cancer, especially the prostate type of cancer, and boost our immunity. The sodium in the tomatoes can help maintain a proper water balance in our body. Sodium also enhances the integrity of both the liver and kidney, keeping them healthy.

Recipes with tomatoes can be found on pages 60, 92, 102, and 134.

Thyme

Thyme is an all-time favorite herb of Joy, my baby sister. When she was experiencing congestion, she juiced 12 ounces of thyme and 1 lb. of small carrots. It quickly expelled her thickened mucous. What a transformation and relief! Thyme may also be beneficial if you are experiencing a sore throat. It contains a small amount of iron, a mineral responsible for transporting oxygen from the lungs to our cells, thereby providing us with vital energy, but we don't have to wait to be weak before adding thyme to our daily diet!

Recipes with thyme can be found on pages 123, 131, and 141.

Turnip Greens

Turnip greens are what I call ageless nutrients. They have an amazing amount of antioxidants known to block the processes that lead to cancer. They contain essential amino acids which are essential to building muscles, blood, and organs, thereby rejuvenating our cells properly. The essential amino acids are important in regulating the level of our mental awareness. I will now discuss the one favorite of mine—methionine, one of the essential amino acids that cleanses and regenerates our kidney and liver cells. It also can be employed as a natural tranquilizer, almost putting you in a state of meditation. And Heaven knows how wonderful it is to have peace within oneself.

A recipe with turnip greens can be found on page 93.

Turnip Roots (see Turnip Greens)

Ugu Leaves

Ugu leaves can help keep excess weight off. It contains nutrients to promote a healthy heart, arteries, and

Juicing For Your Soul

strengthens the immune system. It can also promote rapid wound healing and helps your body slow down the aging process. Ugu leaves contain the vitamin B_{12}, a crucial element to healthy cell division, energy production, and protein metabolism, which are very important to the immunity and the health of our nervous system. If ugu leaves (or kale) have one greatest benefit, it is the ability to supply your body all the calcium it needs to make you feel young and full of vigor, regardless of your real age. Ugu leaves can be found in Nigeria.

A recipe with ugu leaves can be found on page 162.

Watermelons
Watermelons are 100 percent nutritious water. They are closely related to water in that they transport and regulate all the nutrients throughout the body. Due to the high water content of the melon, it is also beneficial in eliminating waste materials and toxins from the body. Watermelons are full of natural vitamins and minerals, as well as essential amino acids. They are very high in pro-vitamin A, an important element for good vision, strong bones, antiviral infection, and skin. One of the essential amino acids in the watermelon is threonine, which stimulates the production of enzymes and digestion by disposing potential carcinogens. The bottom line about watermelons is the fact that they contain so many rich nutrients that may erase many of the signs of aging.

A recipe with watermelons can be found on page 153.

Yams (Sweet Potatoes)
Yams are one of the most nutritious vegetables with more vitamin A content than carrots. They also contain fiber and potassium. The fiber in the sweet potatoes will remove

Juicing For Your Soul

debris from your digestive tract and prevent colon cancer. The vitamin A has the ability to slow down or even prevent the onset of age-related diseases such as heart disease and cancer. The potassium in the yam will help tone the muscles, firm the skin, and promote overall beauty. It can also help restore a high energy level by removing wastes that clog your cells, blood tissues, and organs.

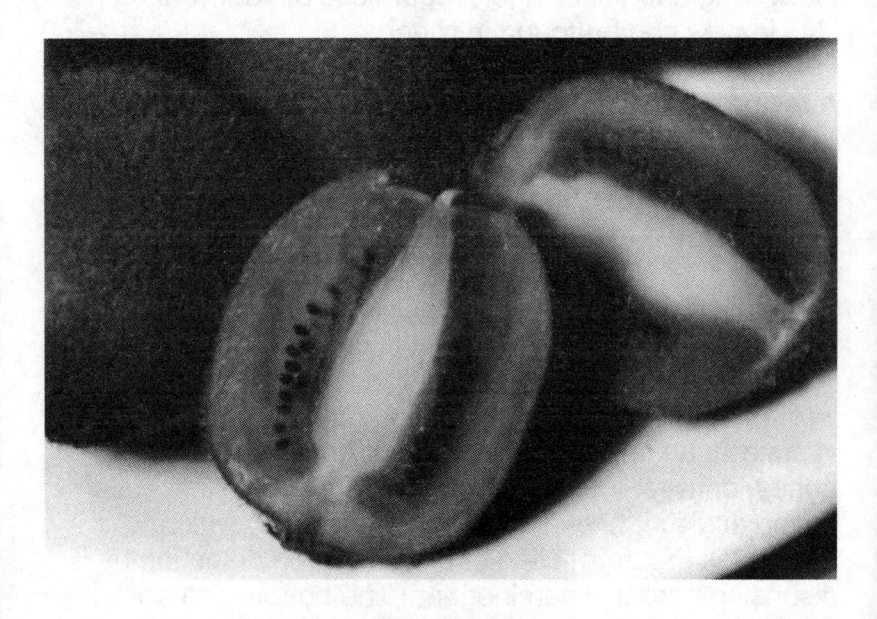

Kiwi Fruit

*Expressing an admiration of love is
the glue of human sweetness*

Juice to Gain Weight

Ingredients	Instructions
1 pineapple (preferably the green one for high content of chlorophyll) 3 apricots 1 pint strawberries	Twist the leaves off of the top of the pineapple and discard them. Wash, scrub, and rinse the pineapple. Cut the pineapple into 2-inch thick rounds and then into strips. Wash all the other ingredients as well. Next, cut the apricots in half and remove the pits. Slice them into small pieces. Remove the green cap from the strawberries. Begin juicing all the ingredients.

Serves 3. Drink immediately.
Very delicious drink! You will find the results quite impressive.

Nutritional Highlights:

Vitamin A can be found in apricots, which is an excellent remedy for healing gastrointestinal ulcers. Apricots contain potassium, a good mineral for stamina. Both strawberries and pineapples are rich in vitamin C, an essential vitamin for building a strong immune system and also helpful in protecting against infection. All of these fruits are full of vitamins and minerals to help energize, as well as support the internal balance the body needs to perform at its peak level. Pineapples are also a great source of bromelain, an enzyme that helps digestion.

Juice to Maintain Kidney

1 whole papaya (preferably a large size or use 2 medium ones)	Using a hard brush, place papaya under running water and scrub for 5-7 minutes. Then slice papaya into 6 sections, making sure the seeds are intact. Begin juicing with both the skin and seeds intact.

Serves 1. Drink immediately.
What a delicious drink full of nutrients! This drink is so easy to make, you can actually close your eyes while making it.

Nutritional Highlights:

Papaya contains vitamin A, an important element for healing the urinary tract and immune system. It also contains vitamins C and E which are both excellent remedies for bowel disorders and indigestion.

Sit down as a stranger…leave as a friend.

Juice to Clean the Internal Cells

1 lb. fresh spinach 1 lb. carrots	Soak the spinach in a big basin full of water for 5 minutes to get rid of the dust, sand, or any other particles. Then wash thoroughly at least 12 times, changing the water until the final rinse water is clear. Scrape off the skins of the carrots, wash thoroughly clean, and cut off the end tips. Cut the carrots in halves, if needed. Proceed juicing.

Serves 2.
Serve immediately and enjoy the experience of "real" juice.

Nutritional Highlights:

Spinach contains coenzyme Q_{10}, a substance that plays a very important role in producing energy in every cell of the body. It helps circulation and stimulates the immune system. Spinach also contains protein which is excellent for repairing muscles in the body. Carrots contain beta carotene and phosphorous. The beta carotene, which is actually vitamin A, promises to be the prevention of some cancers, particularly to those related to cigarette smoking. Phosphorous is an extremely important mineral for the kidney to function at an optimal level and converts food to energy.

Note: A deficiency of phosphorous can lead to fatigue. And if one lacks energy, you become inactive and cell problems begin.

Juice to Cleanse the Liver

½ lb. beets, or if you're like me, you will use 1 lb. 1 lb. radishes	Peel off the skin of the beets. Then wash them before and after cutting them into narrow wedges. Cut off the tops of the radishes. Using a brush under running water, scrub the radishes until thoroughly clean, making sure there are no dark or dirt spots on them. Cut the radishes in halves and then proceed juicing.

Serves 1.
Deliciously alluring!!!

Nutritional Highlights:

Beets contain potassium, an important mineral that helps the body excrete excess sodium and move nutrients via the cell walls. Radishes contain magnesium and potassium. The magnesium helps prevent kidney stones, so you can see why it is important for cleansing the liver.

Note: Cleaning the liver ducts is the most powerful procedure that you can do to improve your body's health. Cleansing the liver dramatically improves digestion, which is the basis of your whole health. You can expect your allergies to disappear the more you cleanse your liver. You have more energy and an increased sense of well-being.

Stay balanced. Simplicity, patience, and compassion.

Juice for Premenstrual Syndrome

1/4 lb. rosemary 1 lb. asparagus	Wash all ingredients thoroughly. You need not discard anything from these vegetables and herbs, but wash them thoroughly. Begin juicing.

Serves 1. Drink immediately.
Quite satisfying!

Nutritional Highlights:

Asparagus contains a high amount of calcium, a nutrient that prevents muscle cramps. Calcium is also excellent in preventing cardiovascular disease and lowers cholesterol levels. Rosemary is an herb that is high in essential oils and an excellent remedy for headache and menstrual cramps.

Note: From the teen years through menopause, most women experience complex changes that may drastically affect their health. This juice will help women be their best at every stage of life.

Fighting is the lowest form of human behavior.

Juice for Strong Bones & Preventing Hemorrhaging in Pregnant Women

½ lb. alfalfa sprouts 1 whole purple cabbage	Use a biodegradable natural cleanser along with water to get rid of any pesticides on the vegetables. Wash the vegetables at least 21 times. Cut the cabbage into small sections. Begin juicing.

Serves 2.
Drink immediately right after juicing to avoid losing any of the nutrients. Enjoy!

Nutritional Highlights:

Both alfalfa sprouts and cabbage contain vitamin K, a necessity for strong bones. It can also prevent osteoporosis. Vitamin K can help to prevent or reduce hemorrhaging. Some doctors even give vitamin K to expectant mothers for the sake of newborn infants. Cabbage contains a high amount of sulfur, a nutrient that disinfects the blood and is excellent for structural integrity of the skin.

Note: Vitamin K may increase resistance to infection in children.

Live royally.

Juicing For Your Soul

Juice for Aneurism Symptoms

1/4 lb. kale 2 lbs. asparagus	Wash all produce thoroughly. You may want to purchase a biodegradable liquid at your health food store to get rid of any chemical spray on the vegetables. Simply begin juicing the kale and asparagus in no particular order, using common sense.

**Serves 2. Drink immediately.
You should feel this go through your blood stream in an instant.**

Nutritional Highlights:

Asparagus contains amino acid. It helps the bowels and soothes the nervous system. Kale, on the other hand, relieves constipation. Both of them produce high amounts of copper which is good for the proper absorption of the iron in our body.

**The law of Karma is so true,
that we reap what we soweth.**

Juice for Removing Mucus

1 whole large red onion or 1 lb. green onions (scallions) 1 lb. carrots	If you use the red onions, just peel off the skins and cut into halves in order to fit into the hopper. And if you use the scallions, just cut off the end portion. Scrape off the skin of the carrots and cut off both end tips. Wash all ingredients before juicing.

Serves 2. Drink immediately. Enjoy!

Nutritional Highlights:

Onions contain high amounts of sulfur, an important element for protecting against the harmful effects of pollution. Sulfur also protects the intestinal walls. Carrots contain the vitamin B complex, an essential element for maintaining good health.

TIPS: Heat and moisture destroy the sulfur.

One who damages the character of another, damages his own.

Juicing For Your Soul

Juice for the Good Life

3 oranges 3 pears, preferably firm and hard, not overripe.	Remove the outer skin of the oranges with a knife, but leave the white pith and membrane intact. Wash the oranges after removing the skin and before cutting. Cut your oranges into halves, set aside. Next, wash your pears thoroughly. Remove the seeds and cut into halves or small enough to fit the juice hopper. Begin juicing.

Serves 2.
Deliciously tasting.

Nutritional Highlights:

Oranges contain natural sugar and zinc. Zinc is an essential mineral which may help prevent acne. Pears contain a high amount of potassium which helps regulate nervous and muscular irritability. So, if you're a nervous wreck, you definitely should drink a glass of this weekly.

Treat yourself royally.

Juice to Retain Sense of Smell & Taste

1 whole honeydew *This is so easy to do.*	*Scrub honeydew under running water for at least 3 minutes, using a hard brush and a biodegradable natural cleanser to get rid of any pesticides.* *Cut into small pieces.* *Proceed juicing.*

Serves 2. Drink immediately.
What a deliciously scrumptious juice, naturally tasty, and naturally digestible.

Nutritional Highlights:

Honeydews are high in zinc, a mineral that allows acuity of taste and smell. Zinc is also needed for nerves.

TIP: Drink two glasses every day for at least a month.

It's a terrible thing and unhealthy that somebody who's done well and is in a leadership role does not take the responsibility to help someone else.

Juice for Healthy Hair

2 lbs. of asparagus	Wash all ingredients thoroughly.
1 lb. of Brussels sprouts	You may cut the Brussels sprouts into halves before putting them through the juicer hopper, just in case they are too large to fit in.
	Begin juicing.

Serves 1.
Drink immediately to avoid losing the nutrients.
Don't expect this drink to taste great, but the result of drinking the juice is certainly worth the taste!

Nutritional Highlights:

Asparagus contains vitamin B_2 (riboflavin) which facilitates the use of oxygen by the tissues of the hairs, as well as eliminating dandruff. Riboflavin is also the essential building block of melanin production. Brussels sprouts contain protein which provides the body with energy and it is needed for the production of hormones.

Note: Following my healthy hair recipe will enable you to achieve the healthy hair you desire while keeping hair soft, supple, and youthful looking.

May the human race learn to share their joys, and not their miseries.

Juice for Acute Anxiety Symptoms

4 broccoli florets with the stems	Slice your broccoli florets and stems into strips, if you desire.
3 or 4 cloves of garlic	Wash all ingredients including the garlic.
1/4 lb. catnip leaves	You may also want to wrap the garlic inside the catnip leaves.
	Begin juicing.

Serves 1.
Here's to peace and harmony!

Nutritional Highlights:

Catnip leaves contain biotin, essential oils, inositol, and folic acid. These nutrients are excellent properties in helping relieve anxiety, digestion, and sleep disorders. Garlic has healing properties such as magnesium and manganese which lowers blood pressure and improves circulation. Broccoli is actually one of my favorite vegetables of all time. Broccoli has a very high amount of calcium, an essential mineral for maintaining a regular heartbeat and nerve impulses. A deficiency in calcium can lead to hypertension, nervousness, depression, and hyperactivity.

"So many people are so primitive that the only thing that covers them up is their latest technology," says my Uncle Cyril.

Juicing For Your Soul

Juice for Indigestion

5 large apples 1 small lemon or lime Handful of sage leaves	Wash and scrub your apples and lime. Pour the sage leaves into a strainer and wash thoroughly under running water several times. Cut the apples, take out the seeds, and cut both halves. Cut the limes into pieces. Begin juicing.

Serves 1!
Here's to a flat stomach!!!

Nutritional Highlights:

Apples are an excellent source of fibrous bulk. They contain several types of fiber, including soluble fiber and pectin. This increases the size of our stools, which then pass onto the colon and trigger natural bowel contractions. Sage leaves contain flavonoids and resin. They stimulate the digestive tract. Limes contain potassium, a vital mineral for a proper muscle contraction.

Note: A healthy digestive system not only helps us feel more comfortable, but enables our bodies to absorb the nutrients we need to live. No matter what your digestive needs, this juice can help.

Spiritual enlightenment does not occur in just a singular moment, but is a gradual, evolutionary, lifelong pilgrimage.

Juice to Relieve Allergies

1/4 lb. dandelion 1/4 lb. peppermint leaves 1/4 lb. spinach	Please, please, please, thoroughly wash all ingredients at least 50 times by placing them all into the strainer under running water. Begin juicing.

Serves 1.
Drink immediately to avoid losing the essential nutrients. This is not the best tasting drink, but it certainly does the job.

Nutritional Highlights:

Spinach contains coenzyme Q_{10}, an important nutrient for improving oxygenation and the immune system. It is a powerful antioxidant and beneficial for people with allergies. Dandelions contain zinc, a vital mineral for a healthy immune system and healing of wounds. Peppermint leaves are a good source of manganese, an important element for healthy nerves and blood sugar regulation. A deficiency of manganese could lead to hearing problems, memory loss, tremors, and pancreatic damage. A deficiency in coenzyme Q_{10} can cause diabetes and muscular dystrophy.

Great health transcends generations.

Juice to Fight Bacteria

3 lbs. fresh red tomatoes	Wash all ingredients thoroughly.
A handful of fresh basil	Slice the tomatoes into narrow sections.
	Begin juicing by first adding the tomatoes into the juicer, followed by the basil.

Serves 2.

What a treat!!! This is so easy to make, you can even close your eyes while preparing this juice.

Nutritional Highlights:

Tomatoes contain sulfur, a mineral that disinfects the blood and helps the body to resist bacteria. Sulfur also protects against toxic substances. Basil, this herb is considered tonic for good spirit and for melancholy.

Your path must be the pursuit of truth, goodness, and beauty.

Juice to Control Migraines

10 medium size oranges	Wash before and after peeling the oranges.
	Peel the outer skins. Then wash. Slice each orange into 4 sections, leaving the white rinds and seeds intact.
	Begin juicing.

Serves 2.
Delicious and soothing!

Nutritional Highlights:

Oranges contain a great amount of phosphorus, essential for contraction of the heart muscle. A deficiency in phosphorus can lead to symptoms such as anxiety and irritability which could lead to a headache.

I do not believe we can do great things for all, but we can do small things with great love.

Juice for Weight Loss

1 big purple cabbage weighing at least 2 lbs 2 fresh limes	After thoroughly washing all the ingredients, slice the cabbage into narrow wedges. Slice the limes into small pieces. Begin juicing immediately.

Serves 1.
It should be drunk within minutes. This is not the best tasting juice, but this juice is so effective, you will feel the difference!

Nutritional Highlights:

Cabbage contains vitamin B5, also known as pantothenic acid, a property that helps to convert fats, carbohydrates, and proteins into energy. Limes are rich in vitamin C, an element for keeping internal cells healthy.

TIP: A deficiency of pantothenic acid may actually cause fatigue. And what happens when fatigue sets in? You're not able to move around like you'd love to.

Juice for a Backache

1/4 lb. alfalfa sprouts 3 lbs. carrots	Thoroughly wash the alfalfa sprouts under fast running water at least 25 times. Trim the carrots. Cut off both top and end tips. Then cut them into pieces. Put the alfalfa sprouts into the juice machine first and use the carrot to push the alfalfa sprouts down the pulper.

Serves 1.

Nutritional Highlights:

Carrots contain vitamin C, an essential component for the formation of collagen which holds all the tissues together. It also relieves tension in the back area and an excellent nutrient for strong bones. Alfalfa contains zinc, an important trace element that protects the liver from chemical damage and it is vital for bone formation.

TIP: The following could cause chronic backache: Poor posture, muscle strain, wear and tear of living, improper lifting and walking, calcium deficiency, slouching when sitting, arthritis, bone disease. And believe it or not, lack of proper bowel movement (constipation) may produce back pain. It doesn't take a scientist to figure out that when one does not eliminate the waste in their body, it actually becomes extra weight! My recommendation is to drink about 10 glasses of water daily to keep acidic wastes from accumulating in the muscles and other tissues.

**Achievements without ethics
will lead to disaster.**

Juicing For Your Soul

Juice for Skin and Hair

3 large cucumbers 4 cloves of garlic A handful of spinach	As always, wash all ingredients under running water and scrub the cucumbers with a brush. Peel the garlic. Slice your cucumbers one by one into four sections. Proceed juicing, pushing them into the hopper.

Serves 1.

What a healthy and luminous skin! For best results, start drinking this juice for seven to ten days. This juice is perfect for preventing and treating dry to severely dry skin due to a poor unhealthy, inactive lifestyle.

The pulp is great for facial treatments. Apply and leave on for 15 minutes. Then rinse with tepid water. Follow with your moisturizing lotion. You may squeeze the liquid from the pulp and add to your moisturizing lotion. Shake well.

Nutritional Highlights:

Cucumbers are high in silicon, a necessity for the formation of collagen for bones and connective tissues. Garlic is an excellent herb for building a strong immune system and getting rid of toxins via the skin. Spinach contains protein, an essential for growth and development.

When you are a righteous person, the "Angels" in the universe will protect you.

Juicing For Your Soul

Juice for Insomnia

2/3 oz. sage	Peel off the skin off of the garlic.
3 cloves garlic (more may be used if desired. I usually use about 10, only when' I'm home. Got the picture?)	Wash and scrub the potatoes leaving the skin intact, then dice them into small pieces so they fit into the mouth of the juice machine.
	Wash the sage equally as well.
3 Redskin or purple potatoes	Begin your juicing.

Serves 1. Drink immediately.

Do not try to save or refrigerate for future use. I recommend juicing and drinking this juice two hours before going to bed or trying to get some sleep. Take the phone off the hook. Shut off your TV or radio and lights to avoid any disturbance.
Have a restful sleep!!!

Nutritional Highlights:

Garlic, sage, and potatoes all contain potassium. Lack of potassium can lead to respiratory distress and frequent headaches. And I'm not so sure how anyone with a constant headache could have a good sleep.

Smiles are free, change is good.

Juicing For Your Soul

Juice for Instant Facelift

2 big cucumbers 1 fresh lemon	Again, you'd want to wash both the cucumber and lemon using a biodegradable liquid and water, using a brush to thoroughly scrub them until they are squeaky clean. No residue or anything slimy should be left on them. Begin juicing.

Serves 1.

Drink immediately and fully reap the nutritional medicinal benefits. My day is always magical whenever I drink this particular juice. It's magical because I can see the glow on my face. I always drink this before I make any public appearance, be it my modeling on the stage, a television appearance, or even going to a charitable function.

Nutritional Highlights:

Lemons are full of good nutrition and they are fat and cholesterol free. Very low in sodium. A medium lemon provides 35% of the daily recommended need for vitamin C, which is so important for healthy skin. Cucumbers contain plenty of sulfur which slows down the aging process. It also stimulates bile secretion. Cucumbers also contain potassium which regulates the transfer of nutrients through cell membrane. Deficiency equals excessively dry skin, constipation, and salt retention.

Don't toil with Mother Nature.

Juice for Low Cholesterol

4 peaches 3 apples 1 quart strawberries 2 lemons	Need I say more? Using a soft natural brush to scrub, wash all ingredients with a biodegradable natural cleanser, along with water. Wash at least 50 times or more to get rid of any pesticides or chemicals that have been sprayed on the produce. I'm not sure why some farmers will want to spray any chemicals on foods! Maybe to make it look good, or what? But always remember that all that glitters is not gold! After washing all produce, remove the seeds from the peaches, and core the apples. Cut the apples, peaches, and lemons into small sections. Remove the green tops of the strawberries. Start juicing.

Serves 2.
Drink right after it is juiced. Here's to your heart!

Nutritional Highlights:

Apples contain pectin which reduces the risk of heart disease. Pectin also removes any unwanted metals and toxins. Strawberries contain sodium, a necessary nutrient for sustaining proper water balance and blood, also helps calm the nerves. Lemons contain bioflavonoids which are excellent for relieving pain. Bioflavonoids also promote circulation. Peaches contain carotenoid, an excellent nutrient for enhancing the immune system and protecting the lungs and mucous membranes.

Juicing For Your Soul

Juice for Hemorrhoid Symptoms

3 whole pawpaw (known as papaya in America)	Leave the skin on the papaya.
	Cleanse thoroughly.
They could be green or yellow. The green ones are unripe which may be excellent for juicing, of course. The yellow ones (ripe) are also good for juicing.	Dice into cross sections making sure you leave the seeds intact.
	Then juice little by little, along with the skin and all.

Serves 1.
What a delight!!!

Nutritional Highlights:

Papayas contain a great deal of fiber and potassium. Fiber is needed to lower the blood cholesterol and for normalizing the stool.

The good life is about love, peace, kindness & compassion.

If you miniaturize the world into a village of 1000, 60 people would be North American, 564 would be Asians, 218 would be Europeans, 80 would be Africans, and 68 would be South American. Of the 1000 people, 700 would be illiterate and 500 would be hungry.

Juice to Increase Oxygen

3 whole pawpaw (known as papaya in America)	Leave the skin on the papaya.
They could be green or yellow. The green ones are unripe which may be excellent for juicing, of course. The yellow ones (ripe) are also good for juicing.	Cleanse thoroughly. Dice into cross sections making sure you leave the seeds intact. Then juice little by little, along with the skin and all.

Serves 2.
What an incredible natural way to put oxygen into the body!

Nutritional Highlights:

Oxygen at the cellular level is essential to growth and life, and strawberries contain quite a bit of oxygen molecules. Lack of oxygen in our tissues is the fundamental reason for all degenerative disease. The growth of any cancer cell is a result of lack of proper oxygen. Cancer cannot and will not live in an oxygenated body. Lemon is helpful when one wants to cut down on weight/fat and it adds a wonderful flavor. It has vitamin C which is an antioxidant, helping protect against cancer, including oral cavity, rectum, breast, stomach, esophagus, and pancreas.

**Today will come
but once leave some kindness behind.**

Juicing For Your Soul

Juice for Antiaging (The Double "A"s)
This juice hydrates and fights the effect of aging. I created this drink for today's lifestyle. It's for people on the go, whether you're going to the office or to the park with the children. It doesn't taste good, but it's remarkably effective. You can have visibly smoother, younger-looking, more radiant skin! I'm so certain you'll love the result of what the mirror-magic will do for you!

2 lbs carrots *2 whole beets* *A handful of parsley*	*Cut off the green tips of the carrots, as well as the bottom. Scrape off the skin. Scrub the carrots under running water with a scouring brush and cut into halves. Cut off the skin of the beets and slice into thin sections. Wash the parsley thoroughly. You may want to use a biodegradable natural cleanser to get rid of pesticides and other chemicals.* *Begin juicing.*

Serves 3.
Drink immediately after flowing from the juice machine.
Quite a plethora of nutrients!

Nutritional Highlights:

Carrots are a great source of beta carotene which the body uses to make vitamin A which is essential for slowing the aging process. A deficiency could lead to dry hair and skin. Parsley is excellent for good bowel movement so nothing stays in your stomach and gut causing all sorts of toxins. Beets to me are indispensable. Let's face it. Many people suffer from chronic constipation because of eating on the go or too fast or all the junk food that has no business being in their stomach to begin with. They contain minerals which contribute to brain function at its best. Heaven knows I need this.

Juicing For Your Soul

Juice for Gall Bladder Symptoms

1 lb. beets	*Cut off the green part of the radishes.*
1 lb. radishes	*Peel off the skin of the beets.*
1/4 lb. dandelions	*Wash all produce at least 50 to 55 times under fast running water.*
	Cut into pieces.
	Begin juicing.

Serves 2.

While drinking, you're probably wondering how much should you juice for one person. Anyhow, common sense should indicate to you that you will need to divide the above ingredients into halves.

Nutritional Highlights:

Dandelions contain more potassium than bananas. My wonderful parents, who taught me everything I know, tell me it is a crucial mineral to life. And believe it or not, it contains vitamin C. Beets are full of good nutrients as they contain sodium and magnesium. Radishes contain plenty of potassium, an important mineral for a regular heart rhythm and is good for maintaining a stable blood pressure.

Your spirit equals your age.

Juicing For Your Soul

Juice for Relaxation

In the hustle and hurry that have become so much apart of our lives, it is important to take a moment at the end of each day to relax/unwind. Celery juice and ginger root, with its mild and soothing flavor, will add a peaceful blend to the close of your day.

1 lb. celery **1/4 lb. fresh ginger root**	*Using a hard brush, scrub the celery and ginger root under running water about 20 to 30 times. Cut or slice the ginger root into small pieces. Throw the ginger root into the juicer one by one and use the celery stick to push the ginger root one after the other until all is juiced.*

Serves 1. Drink immediately.
This drink has a tingling taste to it.

Nutritional Highlights:

Celery contains lots of potassium, which is an important mineral for calming the nerves. Ginger root contains manganese, an important trace element for reproductive processes.

TIP: *Apply the pulp to your face with fingers. Let sit for 10 minutes. This encourages renewal of healthier young skin cells. Then rinse with tepid warm water. Apply lotion.*

"Eating good food is a luxury. It is one of the greatest things about life and it is like one of the Seven Wonders of the World," say my siblings.

Juice for Rejuvenation

Our exceptional blend of 100% fresh oranges and peaches, juiced to perfection, results in a consistently rich and satisfying peachy juice experience. Enjoy the wonderful aroma and exquisite taste of our finest juice blend.

6 peaches **10 oranges**	*Wash peaches. Cut the preaches into narrow wedges. Discard the pits. Peel the oranges, making sure you leave on as much white pith as possible. Cut the oranges into four quarters.* *Begin juicing immediately.*

Serves 3.
Chock full of nutrients!!

Nutritional Highlights:

Oranges are rich in Vitamin C and this is an essential antioxidant nutrient needed for the building of collagen, teeth and gum tissue health, and normal functioning of the body's natural defenses. Peaches are full of magnesium, an essential mineral for soothing irritability in the nervous system.

TIP: *You may use tangerines instead of oranges and still acquire the same result and taste.*

People perish for lack of knowledge.

Juicing For Your Soul

Brain Juice

1 whole green pineapple *3 pears*	Remove the top part of the pineapple. Do not in any way remove the skin. Wash and scrub thoroughly under fast running water using a brush. You should also soak the pineapple in water for about 5 to 10 minutes. Then re-wash again. By soaking it for some minutes, this should remove all the sand or particles. Then cut the pineapple into cross length strips. Wash your pears as well until squeaky clean, also under fast running tap water, using a brush to scrub them. Cut the pears into halves. Remove the seeds. Proceed juicing beginning and ending with the pineapples.

Serves 2.

Nutritional Highlights:

Manganese is a mineral that is found in pineapple and it has a significant contribution to the brain functions. Pears are rich in iron and one of the functions in the body to produce hemoglobin. It also produces oxygen of the red blood cells.

TIP: The brain has a remarkable capacity for memory and activity, but it needs a constant flow of oxygen and nutrients. It depends on glucose as an energy source.

Life is too short and love is rare.

Longevity Juice

2 pints blueberry *4 apples*	*Pour the berries into a strainer and wash under running water until you feel they are thoroughly clean.* *Using a hard brush, wash the apples under running water until clean.* *Then core the apples.* *Begin juicing the apples first and the berries last.*

Serves 2.
What fantastic health ahead of you!

Nutritional Highlights:

Blueberries contain antioxidants, which keep the capillary walls very strong. It also strengthens the collagen and is excellent for antiaging. Apples are one of the greatest fruits on earth for mankind. They are excellent for flushing the kidneys and promoting a good digestive system.

Note: *The goal of the juice here is to provide you with balanced good health, reduce harmful toxins and impurities, cleanse the blood, and promote greater energy.*

My parents once said to me that the eyes are the windows to your health, revealing much about your nutrition levels.

Juicing For Your Soul

Juice for Chronic Anxiety

A handful of peppermint leaves	Trim the carrots, cutting off the lower and upper tips.
1 lb. carrots or 8 carrots	Wash the carrots, garlic and the peppermint leaves.
6 cloves of garlic	Begin juicing.

Serves 1.
Here's to your relaxation!!!

Nutritional Highlights:

Peppermint has a relaxing effect on the muscles. They contain essential oils, which enhance digestion by increasing stomach acidity. It eases anxiety and tension. Garlic, when juiced at least 3 times a week, will reduce blood pressure as well as reduce blood cholesterol. Carrots contain pro-vitamin carotene that is transformed by the body into vitamin A. These two elements destroy cancer-causing problems, and guard against heart disease and stroke, as well as lowering cholesterol levels.

"When people find love and happiness in life, they become content, hence the less drama they inflict on the world," says my brother Franklin.

Juice for Sunday Morning

3 kiwis 2 fresh lemons 3 oranges 3 carrots 6 apples 3 peaches	Remove the skins from the kiwis, oranges, and the carrots. Leave the skins on the lemons, peaches, and the apples. Wash all the fruits and vegetables thoroughly. Cut all ingredients into bite-sized pieces. Please, discard the pit in the peaches. Core the apples as well. Start juicing all ingredients.

Serves 4.

Enjoy! What a flavorful and healthful juice right at your fingertips. It's a great way to start the day with something natural.

Fruits and vegetables provide you with natural roughage, complex carbohydrates, vitamins, and minerals that will lower the risk of your likelihood to a heart attack.

Nutritional Highlights:

Peaches contain lots of potassium, which is crucial for a healthy nervous system. A deficiency in potassium may lead to constipation. Lemons are rich in bioflavonoid, which helps in strengthening weak capillaries. Oranges contain inositol that is vital for reducing cholesterol. Inositol helps remove fats from the liver. When there is low inositol in the body, one can experience high blood cholesterol, mood swings, arteriosclerosis, and constipation. Kiwi fruits contain vitamin C that detoxifies many harmful substances and plays a key role and protects the immune system. Apples contain potassium, which aids in proper muscle contraction. A deficiency can lead to nervousness, high cholesterol levels, and insomnia, which are good for muscle contraction.

Juice for Diminished Appetite

4 oranges *2 lbs. carrots*	*Peel the oranges. Scrape off the skin from the carrots using a carrot peeler. Cut the end and top off the carrots. Wash your produce thoroughly. Slice the oranges into halves.* *Proceed juicing.*

Serves 2.
Deliciously satisfying!

Nutritional Highlights:

Oranges are high in the mineral called copper. Copper is essential for strong bones. It is also needed for energy. Lack of copper or deficiency can lead to such symptoms as weakness. Carrots have a high content of the vitamin B_3. This vitamin is needed for lowering high cholesterol, improving circulation and certainly calming the nervous system.

Act + Act = a certain act of natural consequences.

Juicing For Your Soul

Contaminated Food? Try This Juice

4 cloves of garlic already peeled 4 large cucumbers	Do not peel off the skin of the cucumbers. Cut your cucumbers in halves. Begin juicing, making sure the seeds in the cucumbers are intact.

Serves 2. Drink immediately.

Nutritional Highlights:

Garlic contains sulfur, a strong weapon that will destroy almost any bacteria. It is also useful for strengthening the immune system. Garlic is an excellent aid against bacterial infections. Cucumbers have a good source of choline which helps regulate the gall bladder and reduces too much fat in the liver.

Don't be a slave to material things.

Juicing For Your Soul

Juice for Diabetes Symptoms

½ lbs. string beans or pea pods	All that needs to be done to the beans here is to thoroughly wash them.
3 cloves of garlic	Using a carrot peeler, trim or scrape the skin off of the carrots, and cut both tips off of the carrots.
½ lb carrots	Peel skin off the garlic. Wash all the produce.
	Begin juicing starting with the beans. You may want to use the carrot to push the greens down the hopper, and add your garlic one by one.

Serves 2. Enjoy!

Nutritional Highlights:

Beans contain all the vitamin B complex which will strengthen the blood vessels. Beans also have a high content of magnesium, a mineral necessary for enzymes in producing energy. It also has impact in balancing carbohydrate and mineral metabolism." I can't place enough emphasis on garlic as it lowers blood pressure and reduces the risk of so many other diseases.

Yesterday was all we have.

Juice for Healthy Gums

3 plums 3 kiwis 6 large oranges	Wash all the fruits. Remove the pits from the plums. Peel off the skin from both the kiwis and oranges. Cut your plums, kiwis, and oranges in halves. Begin juicing.

Serves 2.
Deliciously satisfying!!!

Nutritional Highlights:

Healthfully speaking, plums contain a startling amount of nutrients. Many nutrition experts consider plums to be the "perfect food." Vitamin C can be found in kiwis and it also contains antioxidants and protects the gum and makes it strong. Oranges contain vitamin C as well which heals wounds faster.

Life without mercy and compassion is like climbing Mt. Everest without oxygen.

Juicing For Your Soul

Juice for Strong Muscles

8 carrots *1/4 lb. ginger roots (fresh)* *1/4 lb. spinach*	*Using a carrot peeler, scrape the skin off of the carrots.* *Wash all ingredients thoroughly with a brush under fast running water.* *Cut carrots in halves, dice the ginger roots.* *Proceed juicing all ingredients.*

Serves 2.
Here's to healthy muscles.

Nutritional Highlights:

Spinach has a rich source of protein, dietary fiber, and iron. Protein is essential for maintaining a proper acid in the body. Fiber, on the other hand, is necessary for optimum health by lowering cholesterol. Supporting a healthy heart is truly a necessity that is great for your health. Iron, on the other hand, is a necessary mineral that increases energy and alertness, and boosts the immune system. Ginger roots contain a rich source of folic acid, a necessity for stimulating the bowel movement. Carrots, of course, do have a high amount of the C vitamin useful for building strong bones.

Never deny another person a true happiness in life.

Juice for High Blood Pressure

2 lbs. grapes, preferably the dark ones/red, or purple colors with seeds in them. 8 tangerines	Thoroughly wash the grapes at least 20 times to get rid of all the chemicals sprayed on them. Peel off the outer colored rinds of the tangerines. Leave the seeds intact as the juicer will expel them with the fiber. Cut the tangerines into different segments. Begin juicing immediately.

Serves 2. Delicious!!!

Nutritional Highlights:

Both grapes and tangerines have high contents of potassium which is known to help eliminate accumulated salt from the tissues. Tangerines are also full of vitamin C which helps prevent scurvy.

Always use the word 'impossible' with the greatest caution.

Juice for Removal of Toxins

4 lbs. cherries, pitted 1 whole lemon 3 apples	Wash the cherries before removing the pits inside of them. The easiest way I know to remove the pits is to cut the cherries in half and then remove the pit. Wash the apples thoroughly and core them. Discard the seeds and cut them into halves. Wash the lemon before slicing into 4 sections. Proceed juicing.

Serves 2. Enjoy!
What an incredibly yummy taste. It's quite colorful as well.

Nutritional Highlights:

Cherries not only add excellent flavor to just about any other fruits, they are also a source of rich nutrients. Cherries reduce uric acid levels in the body. My father loves what cherry does to him, so he eats 4 lbs. within a day!!! Cherries also contain iron, a requirement for a healthy immune system and for energy production. Lemon contains bioflavonoids which are powerful phytonutrients that nourish the body's cells, tissues, and organs while providing the powerful antioxidant properties that fight damage caused by aging, pollution, and harmful chemicals. Apples contain high amounts of vitamins that are needed by the body for normal growth and tissue maintenance.

Money is a thing of luxury. Good taste is innate.

Juice for the Common Cold

5 broccoli florets with the stems A handful of peppermint leaves 8 carrots	Wash all the ingredients thoroughly. Cut the broccoli florets and the stems into pieces. Using a carrot peeler, peel off the skin of the carrots. Then re-wash all produce again. Cut the carrots into pieces. Begin juicing.

Serves 2.
Drink immediately to avoid the vitamin C dissipating. Enjoy! Drink several glasses of this juice daily until cold is gone.

Nutritional Highlights:

Broccoli contains the mineral selenium which stimulates immune cells that engulf and digest bacteria and other infectious invaders. Carrots contain vitamin C which bolsters the body's defenses to help fend off colds, flu, and other infections. A strong, resilient immune system is your best bet for thwarting cold and influenza germs. Vitamin C lessens the risk of catching cold. Peppermint leaves also contain vitamin C, another essential for building strong mucous membranes.

There's nothing greater in life than loving and being loved.

Juice for Memory Enhancement

2 large red or green bell peppers 6 stalks of celery 2 large cucumbers	Cut off the top of the bell peppers. Using a brush, scrub and wash all ingredients one by one under fast running water until no residue is left. Cut both your peppers and cucumbers into strips. Begin juicing in no particular order.

Serves a family of 3. Drink immediately.
Here's a toast to the good life!

Nutritional Highlights:

Peppers are a great source of silicon and vitamin C. In particular, the abundance of phytonutrients in the peppers, in addition to their vitamin and mineral content, account for memory enhancement. Celery contains all the vitamin B complex and are important for healthy brain function. Cucumbers, on the other hand, contain a mineral called sulfur which is known to keep the aging process at a slow rate.

Don't share your problems unless you're willing to listen to someone else's problem.

Juice for Arthritis

2 firm ripe pears 3 large apples 1 lb. Golden Globe grapes (seeded)	Wash and core the apples. You may want to peel the apples if they look slimy or have pesticides on them. Scrub and wash the pears and grapes as well. Remove the seeds from the pears before juicing. Do not remove the seeds from the grapes as they contain important nutrients. Little by little, run the ingredients through the juicer.

Serves 2. Drink immediately.
Here's to a taste treaty!!! This drink is great for dinner parties or get-togethers; then toasts the event.

Nutritional Highlights:

Both pears and apples contain the mineral called boron known to build strong bones and muscles. They nourish the body's cells and regulate the production of hormones and other substances that are vital to good health. Grapes are rich in potassium, a mineral necessary for strengthening and regulating the heart.

Develop a value that a relationship is for life.

Juicing For Your Soul

Just Diagnosed With Symptoms of Cancer? Try This Uplifting Juice

2 lb. carrots 1 lb. Swiss chard 3 cloves garlic	Peel the carrots and cut off both ends. Wash all ingredients under fast running water. Peel off the skin of the garlic. Cut your carrots vertically. Begin juicing.

Serves 2. Enjoy.

Nutritional Highlights:

Swiss chard contains vitamin A, a powerful antioxidant that enhances the immunity as well as protecting the body from bacteria. Vitamin A is also needed for tissue repair. Carrots also contain antioxidant nutrients such as vitamin C and beta carotene which have powerful anticancer agents by promoting the production of interferon in the body. Garlic is great for enhancing the immune system and as well as removing toxins from the internal cells.

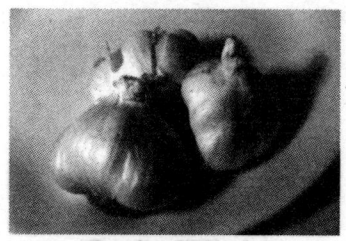

Garlic (Whole)

My parents once said to me that travel is the favorite indulgence of the civilized human being.

Juice for Symptoms of Anemia

½ lb. spinach 4 cloves of garlic 1 lb. burdock root	Wash your spinach thoroughly, making sure there is no sand or dirt left on it. Wash at least 20 times in a strainer under fast running water. Peel the burdock root. Wash thoroughly along with the garlic. Cut the burdock root into medium pieces. Proceed juicing.

Serves 3. Enjoy life!

Nutritional Highlights:

Spinach has an abundance of folic acid, an important nutrient for white blood cells and the immune system. Daily intake of this juice may prevent anemic problems. Garlic contains copper, a mineral used in the healing process and certainly needed for healthy joints. Garlic can be used for a variety of health conditions, including parasites, digestive disorders, and respiratory problems. There are also cardiovascular benefits from drinking this juice. Burdock root contains the mineral zinc which is part of the hundreds of enzymes used by the body for wound repair, vision, fertility, free radical defense.

Looking good isn't good enough.
You have to feel good, too.

Juicing For Your Soul

Juice for Swollen Feet

3 cloves of garlic 4 large celery stalks 3 leaves of collard greens	Wash all your ingredients squeaky clean. Under fast running water, use a vegetable brush to scrub any sand and chemical residue on the celery. Start juicing beginning in this order: Collard greens; then garlic; finally the celery.

Serves 1. Serve immediately.

Nutritional Highlights:

Garlic contains the mineral which act as a disinfectant for the blood. Garlic, by streamlining the body's ability to eliminate waste efficiently, can help. Celery contains all the B vitamins which are good for promoting fluid elimination. Collard greens contain a significant amount of vitamin C, an essential for building strong bones.

Note: Swelling in the extremities is often caused by fluid retention which can be a contributing factor in high blood pressure. You will need to eliminate refined salt in your diet for this juice to have a maximum benefit. Also, try stretching your legs while sitting.

Don't share your misery unless you're willing to share your joy.

Life Enhancement Juice

4 cloves of fresh garlic 1 lb. fresh cilantro 2 large red bell peppers	Wash all ingredients thoroughly. You may use some vinegar. Put the vinegar full strength in a clean spray bottle to safely disinfect both the cilantro and peppers. Just spray the produce. Then really wash and rinse the produce under fast running tap water. Cut your red peppers crosswise into lengths. Begin juicing.

Serves 2. Here's a toast to the good life!

Nutritional Highlights:

Garlic is eminently known to have abundance of antioxidants which have an effect on the immune system because they stimulate white blood cells. Garlic is so rich in sulfur-containing antioxidants, that it is a natural antibiotic, destroying bacteria and yeast directly. One of garlic's immune-boosting qualities makes the brain release serotonin, a neurotransmitter that helps us feel good and stay relaxed. A strong immune system is your first crucial step toward perfect health. Cilantro can help eliminate mercury, toxic metals, or environmental toxins out of the central nervous system for excretion through the urine or feces. Red bell peppers contain silicon which slows the aging process in tissues.

The greatest gift you can give anybody is a laugh.

Good Mood-Lifter Juice

Ingredients	Instructions
2 large red bell peppers 1/4 lb. ginger root (fresh, please) 1 large fresh ripe tomato 6 stalks asparagus	Under fast running water, wash all your produce thoroughly. Using a hard vegetable brush, scrub the peppers, tomato, and ginger root very well. Remove the top part of the peppers. Cut both the peppers and tomato into quarters. Run the peppers, ginger root, tomato, and asparagus through the juicer in this order.

Serves 2. What a tasty treat!

Nutritional Highlights:

Ginger contains manganese and inositol. Manganese is vital in maintaining a balanced blood sugar regulation whereas inositol has a calming effect on the body. Ginger root, in Nigerian medicine, is considered warming and inspiring, and it is used for lifting the spirits. It also lifts depression and induces a meditative state of mind. Tomatoes contain lycopene which is the pigment that gives it the red color. This lycopene fights cancer of the prostrate and can lower the risks of colon and breast cancer, according to Dr. Jelden, —the love of my life—an oncologist here in Ohio. Both asparagus and the red bell peppers have a valuable source of vitamin C which is a premier immune system tonifying vitamin. Vitamin C gives both tremendous protection and support to prevent and help treat colds and other viral and bacterial respiratory infections.

Superior Blood Juice

1 burdock root 1 whole lemon A handful of turnip greens	Wash the burdock root and the greens thoroughly. Using a hard vegetable brush, scrub the lemon under fast running water. Cut both the burdock root and lemon into small pieces. Begin juicing starting with the greens, followed by the burdock root, and then adding the lemon in this order.

Serves 1.
Drink quickly to avoid losing the nutrients. Enjoy your healthy juice!

Nutritional Highlights:

Burdock roots are very important as they are useful in purification of the blood. Turnip greens contain chlorophyll, a trace element. This is a fantastic nutrient that cleanses the red blood cells. Lemons have vitamin P in them, necessary for stimulating bile production.

TIP: Our bloodstream is renewed every 3 months and every 11 months every cell in the body itself If you keep the body clean both internally and externally, how can you get sick? Keep the body clean by eating a diet that continually purifies the body so that you can defy the signs we have come to associate with sickness.

To be peaceful is the highest achievement of the self.

Juice to Relieve Diarrhea

3 large red bell peppers	Wash all produce thoroughly.
1 lb. Swiss chard	Peel the onion.
½ of a small red onion	Remove the top part of the peppers and then re-wash.
	Cut the peppers and onions into small sections.
	Put the onions into the juicer first, then follow with the rest of the ingredients.

Serves 2. Drink immediately.
So colorful and tasty!

Nutritional Highlights:

Both the red peppers and Swiss chard have a high content of beta carotene which is an important antioxidant. Another healing factor of the beta carotene is to protect and heal the lining of the colon. Onions have important nutrients for strengthening a strong immune system.

TIP: Avoid taking laxatives when suffering from diarrhea. Drink at least 9 glasses of water per day.

***We are what we eat, drink,
breathe, think and do.***

Juice for Peace

8 oranges 2 pints of blueberries (fresh, please)	Peel the oranges, leaving on as much white pith as possible. Wash the oranges. Put the berries into a strainer and place under running water, shaking it slightly. Use your hands to wash them as they are very soft. Cut the oranges into quarters. Begin juicing using half of the oranges first and the remainder last.

Serves 3. Drink immediately.

Nutritional Highlights:

Both oranges and blueberries contain vital nutrients of flavonoids and not only do they strengthen connective tissue, but they also are useful for relieving anxiety and stress. Oranges do have some nutrients capable of lowering blood pressure.

A healthy thriving life is as inalienable as anything.

Asthma Symptoms Juice

1 lb. red seeded grapes 6 large oranges	Remove the stems from the grapes leaving everything else intact. Wash thoroughly and set aside. Peel the oranges, leaving on as much of the white membrane as you can. Wash oranges after peeling. Cut the oranges into quarters. Begin juicing starting with the oranges, followed by the grapes.

Serves 2. Consume immediately.
Mmmmm delicious.

Nutritional Highlights:

Grapes contain vitamin A which is needed for the growth and repair of body tissues. It also helps to protect the mucous membranes of the nose, mouth, throat, sinuses and lungs. Grapes are also high in fiber, a necessity—regular elimination of toxins thus maintains a healthy digestive tract. Oranges contain vitamin A as well and the vitamin A has another function which is to protect one against pollution and colds.

Make it a great day.
All day–Everything!

Juice to Relieve Oily Skin

4 oranges 1 pint raspberries	Peel the oranges, leaving the white membrane intact. Wash and then cut into quarters. Pour the berries into a strainer and rinse thoroughly under fast running water. Begin juicing starting with the oranges and ending with the raspberries.

Serves 1. Enjoy!!!

Nutritional Highlights:

Raspberries contain both zinc and selenium. These minerals are key nutrients needed to build healthy skin. Oranges have a wide range of beneficial effects on the circulatory and central nervous systems.

My parents once told me "to live a good life, one should have isolationist mind-set."

Juicing For Your Soul

Juice to Relieve Motion Sickness

1/4 lb. fresh peppermint leaves 2 large apples 3 fresh apricots	Wash all ingredients. Scrub both the apples and apricots with a brush under fast running water. Spray some vinegar to get rid of the pesticides. Core the apples and cut into quarters. Cut the apricots and remove the pits and slice into halves. Begin juicing starting with the apples first, then the peppermint leaves, and then the apricots.

Serves 1. Really delicious!

Nutritional Highlights:

Both apples and apricots have rich sources of the mineral called magnesium. Its role includes the energy production of glucose and neuromuscular contractions. Peppermint leaves strengthen the stomach and cleanse the entire system. They also contain a significant amount of the C vitamin and one of its functions is healing wounds due to the fact that it facilitates the formation of connective tissue in the scar.

TIP: Signs of motion sickness could range from vomiting to severe headaches, dizziness while sailing or traveling in cars. I certainly have had experience with this sickness while sailing with my boyfriend on his boat on our first date. I vomited the whole day. Yikes!

It is your love that will change the world.

Juice to Relieve Carpal Tunnel Syndrome

3 pears 3 peaches 8 tangerines	Soak both the peaches and pears in vinegar, using about 1/4 cup for 5 minutes in cold water. Scrub them under running water, using a brush and mild soap until squeaky clean. Cut off both ends of the tangerines and remove the skin with your fingers or you may use a knife to peel off the skin. Core the pears and cut into quarters. Cut the peaches and remove the seed. Cut the peaches and the tangerines into halves. Begin juicing.

Serves 2. Serve immediately.
What a delightful way to enjoy a friend with this drink.

Nutritional Highlights:

Pears and tangerines are excellent for healing purposes as they both contain vitamin C. The C vitamin's function is to maintain collagen which is a protein that is necessary for the formation of connective tissue in skin, bones, and ligaments. Peaches are one of the most nutritious fruits and are high in potassium, an excellent mineral for regulating the transfer of nutrients to cells. All these fruits are healing food for the whole body.

TIP: Try not using your wrist at all times. Let them relax. Use your whole hand and all of your fingers when holding an object. Try to have good posture. Use arm rests to keep your wrists from over flexing.

Juice for Menopause

16 ounces fresh cranberries (or 2 cups) *3 large pears*	*Wash the pears using a soft brush under fast running water, adding a little vinegar as you clean.* *Place the cranberries into a strainer and rinse thoroughly under cold water.* *Cut the pears into quarters and remove the seeds.* *Then begin juicing.*

Serves 2. Enjoy!

Nutritional Highlights:

Cranberries tend to counter the severity of hot flashes, mood swings, periodic bloating, as well as bladder infections. Cranberries have in them vitamin C which is known for warding off infections from the urinary tract. Pears have megadoses of vitamin B_1 (thiamine) which acts as an antioxidant by protecting the body from degenerative effects of aging.

TIP: *A deficiency of the B_1 vitamin can cause irritability, forgetfulness, and pain.*

There is nothing wrong with money; it's how you acquire it and how you use it once it is acquired.

Mental and Physical Energy Juice

4 oranges 4 apricots, fresh please!	Peel the outer skin of the oranges, leaving on the white pith and membrane.
	Wash the oranges and apricots for at least 5 minutes. Remove the stones from the apricots.
	Cut the oranges into quarters. The apricots may not need to be cut as they are small enough to fit into the juice hopper.
	Beginning with the oranges, start juicing and end with the apricots.

Serves 2. Enjoy!

Nutritional Highlights:

Both oranges and apricots are rich in potassium, a mineral necessary for stimulating the kidneys and regulating the heart beat. Oranges also possess the vitamin B complex which supports the physical and mental energy. Niacin, also known as vitamin B_3 which is part of the B complex, helps maintain cholesterol levels that are already within a healthy range. Apricots has the ability to nourish and strengthen the body.

TIP: A deficiency of potassium could lead to depression and muscular weakness.

**My parents once said to me that
"arrogance, hate and racism are supported by ignorance."**

Juice to Relieve Stomach Ulcer

2 large tomatoes A handful of alfalfa sprouts 1/4 lb. purple cabbage A handful of fresh peppermint leaves	Place both the alfalfa sprouts and the peppermint leaves into a strainer and wash them with your hands under running water until you feel they are clean. Wash the tomatoes with a hard brush under running water. Then wash your cabbage. Cut both the tomatoes and cabbage into quarters. Please, cut off the black top of the tomatoes before juicing. Begin juicing putting in the cabbage first, the tomatoes second, and the peppermint leaves with the alfalfa sprouts in this order, ending with the leaves and sprouts.

Serves 2. Consume immediately. Enjoy!

Nutritional Highlights:

Both tomatoes and alfalfa have a high amount of the vitamin B_3 that is part of the vitamin B complex. The B_3 is needed for stimulating digestion and to support overall vitality. The B_6 vitamins can be found in cabbage, an essential for enzyme production and wound healing. Alfalfa also contains vitamin B_{12}, which is required for normal metabolism of carbohydrates and fats, healthy cell replication, energy metabolism, and nerve and immune function. Peppermint leaves contain a significant amount of vitamin C which is needed for anti infection.

TIP: *The B vitamins are water-soluble; they are continually excreted, and must be constantly replaced.*

Stress Relief Juice

3 large oranges *2 large fresh apples*	*Peel the oranges. Wash and cut into quarters. When peeling the oranges, make sure you leave on as much of the white membrane as possible. Wash your apples under fast running water using a brush. But if you suspect the apples are sprayed with wax or pesticides, peel off the skins. Core the apples and cut into quarters. Remove seeds, please.* *Begin juicing immediately.*

Serves 1. Consume immediately. Enjoy!
What a fabulous way to relieve tension!

Nutritional Highlights:

Oranges contain vitamin C, which is essential to life. Vitamin C contributes to healthy strong bones. Oranges also have a high content of calcium, which is an important mineral responsible for building strong healthy bones and teeth. It also acts as a natural tranquilizer. Apples contain magnesium, a mineral crucial for converting blood sugar into energy. This plays a key role in muscular relaxation and supports the integrity of the arteries and heart.

TIPS TO DE-STRESS: *Take some time for yourself. If you nurture yourself, you'll feel more centered when you deal with daily challenges.*

Gout Relief Juice

1 medium size sweet potato 1/4 lb. fresh dill	Wash all the vegetables thoroughly in water using 2 tablespoons of vinegar. Scrub the potatoes with a hard brush. Cut the potatoes into small pieces. Begin juicing beginning with the potatoes and ending with the dill.

Serves 1.

Nutritional Highlights:

Sweet potatoes contain a high significant amount of vitamin E, an element necessary for removing excessive formation of uric acid. Gout is a type of arthritis characterized by an excess of uric acid. Vitamin E is also important in cellular respiration of all muscles. Dill contains fiber, which is necessary for eliminating internal rubbish, and helps maintain a healthy colon. When you have normal regularity, then there is no room for disease.

TIP: You should try to reduce the amount of your alcohol intake or eliminate it completely if you can, since it stimulates the production of uric acid. If you're a drinker and have gout, you're probably thinking to yourself that life will not be the same without your bottle!!! Gout is caused by a buildup in the body of uric acid which is found in high amounts in animal meats. When the level of uric acid rises to unhealthful levels in the body, it crystallizes, causing sharp needle-like pain.

Enjoy every minute!

Juice for Eczema

3 pears 3 nectarines	Soak both the pears and nectarines in water. Add 2 tablespoonfuls of vinegar to the water. Let soak for 3 to 5 minutes.
	Scrub under running water with a brush.
	Cut the pears into quarters and remove the seeds. Cut the nectarines and remove the seeds as well.
	Begin juicing starting with the pears first and ending with the nectarines.

Serves 2.
Delicious!

Nutritional Highlights:

Both nectarines and pears have high contents of vitamin A and this vitamin is extremely beneficial for clear, healthy skin. Vitamin A is also necessary for preventing dryness of the skin.

TIP: You should refrain from eating chocolates, sweets, fried foods, and all junk foods as they may precipitate the problem more.

Cleanliness is nothing you do in haste.

Juice for Sore Throat

2 mangoes *3 oranges*	*Soak the mangoes in water and add 2 tablespoons of vinegar. Let stand for 5 minutes.*
	Scrub them very hard with a brush under running water. Peel the oranges and then wash.
	Peel the mangoes and remove the seeds.
	Cut the oranges into quarters.
	Begin juicing adding the oranges first, followed by the mangoes.

Serves 2.
Tasty! To truly appreciate the taste of this drink, you really have to possess an instinct of a good taste!

Nutritional Highlights:

Mangoes contain vitamin C which is beneficial for reducing the effects on the body of some allergy-producing substances. Another role of the C vitamin is as an antioxidant, which among other things, keeps capillary walls strong and flexible. The C vitamin also is a powerful anti-inflammatory and immune system stimulant. Oranges have a high content of vitamin A, essential for protecting the mucous membranes of the throat. This same protection helps the mucous membranes in combating the effects of invasive microorganisms and other harmful particles. Mangoes contain a remarkable spectrum of components valuable for human health.

Juice for Headache Relief

2 lbs. of carrots 1/4 lb. fresh ginger root 1/4 lb. fresh peppermint leaves	Scrape off the skin of the carrots. Wash thoroughly in vinegar and water. Use a vegetable brush to scrub the ginger under running water, making sure all the dirt is completely rinsed off. Place both the ginger root and the peppermint leaves into a strainer and rinse thoroughly using your hands. Cut the carrots into halves and dice the ginger root. Begin juicing.

Serves 2.
Drink immediately to avoid losing any of the nutrients.
Enjoy!

Nutritional Highlights:

Peppermint is an herb that contains niacin which is vitamin B_3 and may be helpful for headache sufferers. Ginger root is another great herb that contains inositol which acts like a tranquilizer. Inositol is essential for the growth and survival cells in bone marrow and eye membranes. Carrots also contain vitamin B_3 which plays a role in maintaining a normal dilation of the blood vessels. Niacin is also excellent for maintaining a healthy nervous system.

TIP: If you have repeated headaches, this may signal a serious disorder. You should contact an acupuncturist or a chiropractor. Avoid using salt, chewing gum, tobacco, and wine, as they may cause migraine headaches. Hatred also causes severe headaches. So think of beauty and truth.

Juice for Epilepsy/Seizure Symptoms

1 lb. fresh spinach 1/4 lb. radishes 3 large carrots	Use a brush under running water to thoroughly scrub the dirt off of the radishes. Wash the spinach and the radishes with vinegar and water. Scrape off the skin of the carrots and wash them until squeaky clean. Cut the carrots into halves and cut the radishes if they are too big to fit inside the hopper. Begin juicing.

Serves 2.
Nutritionally correct! Enjoy!

Nutritional Highlights:

Spinach contains a vitamin-like substance called coenzyme Q_{10} necessary for improving brain oxygenation. This is also a powerful antioxidant and may strengthen muscles as well as help in removing molecules that attack healthy cells in the body and leave it vulnerable to disease. Radishes contain magnesium, an essential mineral necessary for proper functioning of the muscles. Carrots also contain important minerals called potassium which is necessary for normal growth. It stimulates the kidneys to eliminate poisonous body wastes.

One has to be grateful to life at all times.

Muscle Cramps Relief Juice

2 large grapefruits 2 pints of raspberries	Peel the grapefruits, leaving on as much of the white membranes as possible. Wash and cut into 4 sections. Pour the raspberries into a strainer and rinse well under water, adding a teaspoon of vinegar. Begin juicing starting with the grapefruits first and ending with the raspberries.

Serves 2. Drink immediately.
Delicious! Enjoy!

Nutritional Highlights:

Raspberries contain magnesium, an important mineral that is involved in many essential metabolic processes including the muscle action. Grapefruits have a high content of calcium which is necessary for normal muscle contraction and stimulation. Calcium, an important mineral, is also needed for the development and maintenance of bone structure and rigidity.

TIP: An imbalance in the levels of calcium and magnesium in the body can result in muscle cramping. Lack of exercise can result in poor circulation and dehydration can lead to muscle cramps. Protecting your bones is one of the most important things you can do for yourself.

Happiness is something that must be cultivated.

Juicing For Your Soul

Juice for Morning Sickness Symptoms

3.5 oz fresh peppermint leaves 1 lb. carrots 1/4 lb. fresh ginger roots	Peel the carrots and cut off both the ends. Cut the carrots into halves so as to fit the pulp into the juicer so it will not do any damage. Wash all the vegetables, adding 2 tablespoonfuls of vinegar. Rinse thoroughly until squeaky clean. Begin juicing.

Serves 1. Enjoy!

Nutritional Highlights:

During times of morning sickness, juicing peppermint leaves will strengthen the stomach as well as providing a soothing stomach. It also contains some trace minerals to help reduce cravings during pregnancy that may be caused by the body's need for more minerals. Ginger root is an excellent remedy for relieving nausea and fever. Ginger root is also used to strengthen and stimulate vital energies while invigorating the whole body. Carrots contain beta carotene which is a precursor of vitamin A, a necessity for building a strong immune system. Beta carotene is a powerful antioxidant, an essential for destroying free radical-causing disease agents and ensures all cells remain healthy.

Life is a gift and it can be taken away any time. You must respect it.

Juice for Burns

8 kiwis 15 tangerines	Peel off the skin of the kiwis and tangerines. You can actually use your fingers to peel off the skins on the fruits. Then wash thoroughly. Start juicing beginning with the tangerines and ending with the kiwis.

Serves 2.

What a grandeur taste! Drink as soon as it has been made. If not, all the essential nutrients will degrade after a while.

Nutritional Highlights:

Kiwis contain significant amounts of vitamin A which is necessary for tissue repair as well as for building strong bones and teeth. Kiwis also contain protein which is necessary to rebuild or replace tissues that no longer function properly. The protein in the kiwis can also maintain optimum growth and great health. Kiwis are very low in calories. Tangerines contain vitamin C which is a powerful antioxidant necessary for healing of burns as well as aiding in the formation of collagen. Tangerines also contain small amounts of folic acid, an important element for mental and emotional health.

TIP: If you have a severe burn such as a third-degree burn, take yourself to the doctor. Drink plenty of water and this juice.

Out of diversity comes happiness.

Juice to Relieve Bladder Infection

1 quart fresh cranberries *2 large grapefruits*	*Peel the grapefruits, leaving on the white membranes.* *Wash the grapefruits after peeling, then cut into quarters.* *Pour the cranberries into a strainer and rinse well under tap water.* *Begin juicing by adding the grapefruits first, then add a handful of the cranberries, and end with the grapefruits.*

Serves 1.
What a delightful and remedious juice!

Nutritional Highlights:

Cranberries contain valuable nutrients that prevent bacteria in the bladder and kidney as well as keeping the entire urinary tract from infection. Cranberries also contain vitamin C, an essential that protects the body from bacterial infection. Grapefruits have a great source of potassium, an important mineral that is essential for the kidneys to maintain their normal serum levels through their ability to filter and excrete fluids.

TIPS: Decrease your intake of salt and refined sugar.

Juicing For Your Soul

Juice to Relieve Heart Disease

8 oranges 4 cloves of garlic	Peel the oranges, leaving on as much white membrane as possible. Place the oranges in a container, adding 3 tablespoons of vinegar. Rinse very well. Then cut into quarters. Peel off the outer skin of the garlic. You may want to wear gloves to avoid the smell lingering in your hands. Begin juicing starting with the oranges first and ending with the garlic.

Serves 2. Enjoy!
Delicious and satisfying.

Nutritional Highlights:

Oranges have vitamin C, an important antioxidant to help fight infection. It protects the lungs from damage and promotes healing. Adequate intake of this juice is essential as it may lower blood cholesterol. Garlic offers a host of benefits. It can reduce the risk of fatal heart attacks. And garlic is also effective in dissolving and cleansing cholesterol from the blood stream.

**By changing ourselves,
we allow the world to change.**

Eye Protection Juice

2 large size grapefruit 5-8 oz. raspberries 4 cloves of fresh garlic (optional)	Peel the grapefruit, leaving the white pith part intact. Wash the grapefruit thoroughly clean and cut into strips. Peel the garlic and put both the garlic and raspberries into a strainer and rinse thoroughly under running water. Begin juicing starting with the grapefruit first, raspberries second, garlic third, and ending with the grapefruit again.

Serves 1.
Tasty and perfect for the eyes!

Nutritional Highlights:

Grapefruit and raspberries are both rich in vitamin C, a powerful antioxidant which provides protection for many of the body's important systems by combating free radicals and oxidants—molecules which damage cells. Vitamin C also contains key nutrients that support the health of the eye itself, increasing the chances of excellent sight. Garlic contains vitamin A, essential for the skin and mucus membranes.

TIPS: Exercise, proper nutrition, compassion, kindness, and positive thinking are essential to maintaining a healthy lifestyle.

Think of beauty and truth.

Juice for Relief of Constipation

4 to 6 cloves of fresh garlic 4 large fresh apples 6 ounces of alfalfa sprouts	Peel off the skin of the garlic. Put both the garlic and the sprouts into a strainer and rinse very well under running water using your hands. Soak the apples in dishwashing liquid for 5 minutes and scrub with brush. Then re-soak the apples with clear water and 1/4 cup of vinegar and wash thoroughly. Core the apples and remove both the stems and the seeds. Cut the apples into quarters. Begin juicing starting with the apples first, then the sprouts, then the garlic, and ending with the apples.

Serves 2. Enjoy!
Must consume immediately to get the full nutritional values.

Nutritional Highlights:

Apples contain high amounts of pectin which is a fiber found under the skin of apples and is important for softening of the stool, thereby providing one with regular bowel movements. Alfalfa sprouts are an excellent herb for preventing stomach problems and very useful for digestion. Garlic contains allicin which gives garlic the smell when crushed and is helpful in stimulating the walls of the intestines.

Be able to laugh at your misfortunes.

Juicing For Your Soul

Juice for Vigor and Vitality

12 ounces blackberries 4 oranges 2 mangoes	Put the berries into a strainer and rinse very well under running water. You may want to add 2 tablespoons of vinegar while rinsing to get rid of any toxic substances. Put the mangoes in water, add 2 tablespoons of vinegar and let soak for 5 minutes. Peel the oranges, leaving as much of the white pith intact as the pith contains important nutrients. Wash and cut into quarters. Scrub the mangoes under fast running water and remove the pit inside. Cut mangoes into small pieces. Begin juicing starting with the oranges first, then the mangoes, then the berries, and ending with the oranges.

Serves 2.
The aroma and color of this drink are deliciously inviting and perfect for listening to jazz or classical music! Optimal health, vitality and energy at your fingertips!

Nutritional Highlights:

Mangoes contain pantothenic acid which is the vitamin B_5 necessary for metabolizing carbohydrates, fats, and protein for the release of energy. Oranges, especially the white part, contain bioflavonoids which strengthens the capillary walls. Blackberries contain potassium, a mineral necessary for keeping the skin healthy and keeping a stable blood pressure. Oranges also contain the vitamin B-complex which influences many different aspects of health.

NOTES: Oxygen is the breath of life and a critical component of your metabolism. It is the catalyst for quick energy.

Juice That May Help Prevent Parkinson's Disease

5 oranges 5 carrots or 1 lb. 3 or 4 cloves of garlic	Oranges should be peeled, leaving the white part intact. Peel off the skin of the carrots, as well as the garlic. Wash all produce thoroughly, adding about 1/4 cup of vinegar. Cut the oranges into quarters. Cut off both tip ends of the carrots. Begin juicing starting with the oranges first, the garlic second, the carrots third, and ending with the oranges.

Serves 2. What opulence!

Nutritional Highlights:

Oranges contain all the vitamin B complex which is important for the normal functioning of the nervous system and are often helpful in bringing relaxation to those who are stressed. Vitamin B1, which is part of the B-complex, helps to prevent the accumulation of fatty deposits in the arteries and is essential for nearly every cellular reaction in the body. Carrots contain niacin, or B3, which can assist in the reduction of high cholesterol and can ease stress and anxiety. Garlic contains vitamin B2 or riboflavin, an essential for improving memory.

Juicing For Your Soul

*NOTES: Parkinson's disease is a slowly progressive disease of the nervous system in which an essential type of nerve cell located in a small part of the brain is destroyed. Chronic constipation may complicate the condition. For treatment of constipation, see **Juice to Relieve Constipation**. Regular exercise of any sort will help with flexibility, mobility, balance, and coordination. Walking, stretching, or using a cycling machine is recommended.*

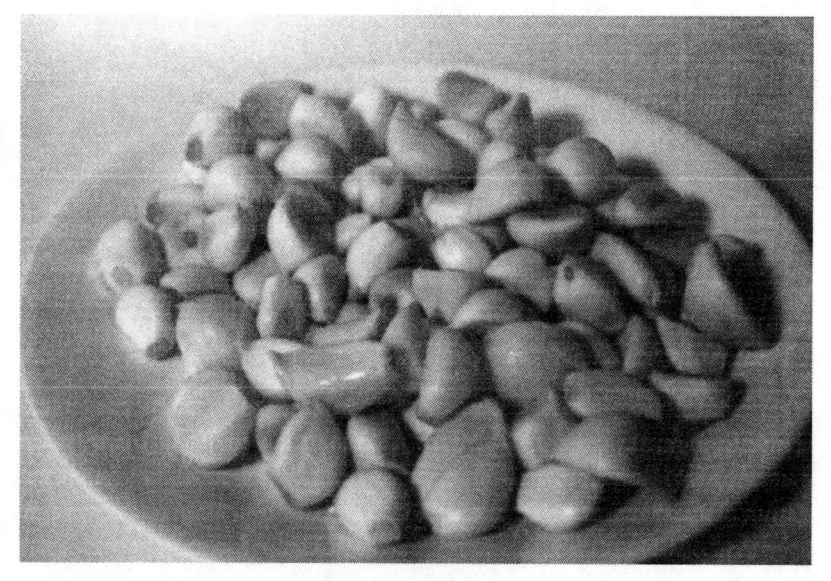

Garlic (Peeled)

"You must not allow the world to take away the joy that they did not give you," says my great, great grandmother.

Juice for Halitosis/Bad Breath

10 oz. fresh parsley 1 bag or 1 lb. radishes 1 whole lemon	Put the parsley into a strainer and rinse very well until squeaky clean. Take a brush and scrub both the lemon and radishes under running water until quite clean. You may add some vinegar while washing. Cut the lemons into 6 pieces. Cut the radishes into halves so as to fit into the hopper. Begin juicing starting with the radishes, then the parsley, then the lemon, and ending with the radishes.

Serves 1. Drink immediately. Enjoy!

Nutritional Highlights:

Parsley is excellent for freshening breath. It contains chlorophyll and is very high in antioxidants. Lemons contain vitamin C which can boost the body's natural immune system, thereby healing both the mouth and gum disease. Vitamin C also fights infections in the body. Radishes are an excellent source of calcium, a mineral for building strong bones and teeth.

NOTES: This juice in not an excuse for not brushing your teeth. Please brush both your teeth, tongue and areola ridge (the upper part of your mouth). Change your toothbrush every two weeks and keep them clean. Store your toothbrush in a cup full of water and 2 tbls. vinegar. Change the water on a daily basis. As a mouth rinse, chew on the pulp of this juice after eating. Spend at least 10 minutes brushing every corner of your mouth and use any bath soap to wash both your upper and lower lips after brushing.

Juice for Hangover Relief

4 quarts or 4 pints of alfalfa sprouts 1 lb. carrots	Scrape off the skin of the carrots and cut off both tips. Wash very well using a soft brush to scrub the carrots. Place the alfalfa sprouts into a strainer and rinse until thoroughly clean. Cut the carrots into halves. Start juicing beginning with the carrots, then the alfalfa sprouts, and ending with the carrots.

Serves 2. What an indulgence!

Nutritional Highlights:

Alfalfa sprouts contain the vitamin B complex which helps maintain a healthy muscle tone. In addition, the B vitamins are necessary for normal functioning of the nervous system. Both alcoholics and hyperactive individuals can greatly benefit from this juice. The vitamin B-complex helps to detoxify the body as well. Carrots are rich in niacin or B3 vitamin which is vital for reducing high cholesterol, as well as to ease stress and anxiety.

TIPS: Do not drink alcohol on an empty stomach. Add some water to your alcohol for dilution purposes. Drink the above juice before drinking alcohol. If you are a small person, like me, you will want to drink just half a glass. Eat plenty of peanuts as they are helpful due to their high content of protein. Please, for heaven's sake, don't drink and drive!

Living as one race is primitive and deceitful.

Juice for Heartburn

1/4 lb. fresh ginger root 4-7 ounces fresh peppermint leaves 1 lb. carrots	Using a scouring brush under running water, scrub the ginger root and wash very clean. Do not peel the skin; just get the dirt off. Put the peppermint leaves on a plate and rinse very well with a teaspoon of vinegar. Scrape off the skin of the carrots and cut off both ends. Dice the ginger into small pieces. Wash the carrots until very clean before juicing. Start juicing beginning with the carrots, leaves, ginger, and ending with carrots.

Serves 1. A yummy juice full of rich nutrients.

Should you need to juice for 2 or more, just double or triple the size portion of the ingredients.

Nutritional Highlights:

Ginger root is used to strengthen and stimulate vital energies while invigorating the whole body. Peppermint is another herb that possesses a soothing effect on the digestive tract and stimulates digestive secretion. Carrots contain vitamin A which is crucial to building a strong internal immune system. And a healthy immune system controls the body's ability to resist infection and recover from illness, which is also crucial to healthy digestion.

Juicing For Your Soul

NOTES: *The following foods should be avoided when heartburn exists: dairy products, fast foods, soft drinks, and coffee. Avoid eating too fast as this is the main culprit.*

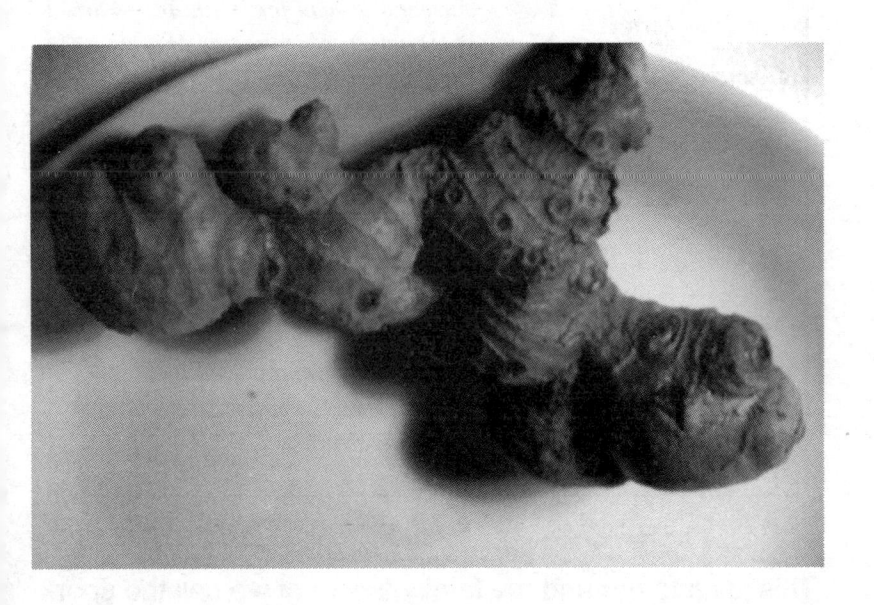

Ginger Root

***Relax and try not to worry.
Take life easy before it takes you.***

Juice for Cardiovascular Activities

8 oz. fresh spinach 1 lb. fresh carrots 4 ounces fresh thyme	In a sink full of water, add 1/4 cup of vinegar and soak for 5 minutes. Wash at least 10 times to get rid of the sand and grit. Scrape off the skins of the carrots and cut off both tips. Wash the carrots very well. Pour the thyme into a small container and rinse well. Cut the carrots if they are too big to fit into the hopper. Start juicing beginning with the spinach, then the thyme, and ending with the carrots.

Serves 2. Enjoy!
This juice to me and my family are what we call the spark of the good life and the energy exchange.

Nutritional Highlights:

Spinach has high amounts of coenzyme Q10,, which plays an essential role in producing energy in the cells. It is a powerful antioxidant with antiviral antitumor properties. It also has heart protective effects as well as potent immune nutrients. Thyme and carrots are both rich in the vitamin B complex responsible for providing the body with energy by aiding in the conversion of carbohydrates to glucose, which the body burns to produce energy.

NOTES: As we become advanced in years, our body's storage of CoQ10 becomes depleted; therefore, it is important that we replace them. Wait 20 minutes before engaging in exercise.

Juicing For Your Soul

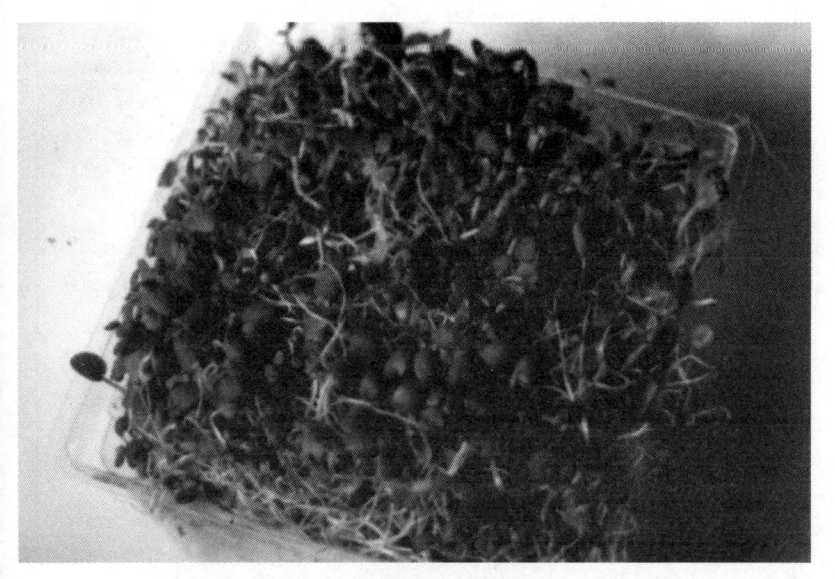

Crushed Alfalfa Sprouts

My parents once said to me, "he who lives by the island should not become an enemy of the sea."

Juice for Muscle Coordination

2 mangoes 1 whole unripe pineapple 4 oz. Fresh sage leaves	In a sink full of water, add 1/4 cup of vinegar and soak both the mangoes and pineapple for 10 minutes. In the meantime, pour the sage in a strainer and rinse well under running water. Set aside. Scrub both the pineapple and mangoes under running water using a mild dish soap detergent and wash thoroughly for about 10 minutes to get rid of all the pesticides and rubbish. Cut the mangoes and remove the large pit inside. Cut off both ends of the pineapple tips and discard them. Cut both the mangoes and the pineapple into strips. You must leave on the outer skin as this contains 95% of the nutrients. Start juicing beginning with the pineapple, then the mangoes, then the sage leaves, and ending with the pineapple.

Serves 3. What a delight!

Nutritional Highlights:

Pineapples are a great source of manganese, a trace mineral which aids muscle weakness by stimulating the transmission of impulses between nerve and muscle and the overall feeling of well-being. Sage, a herb known for ages, is an excellent medicinal remedy that stimulates the central nervous system. It has also been known for ages to heal wounds. Mangoes contain a significant amount of vitamin C. Vitamin C is important for people in the so-called modern age because of its ability to protect us from damage caused by toxic elements in the environment, including heavy metals and chemicals.

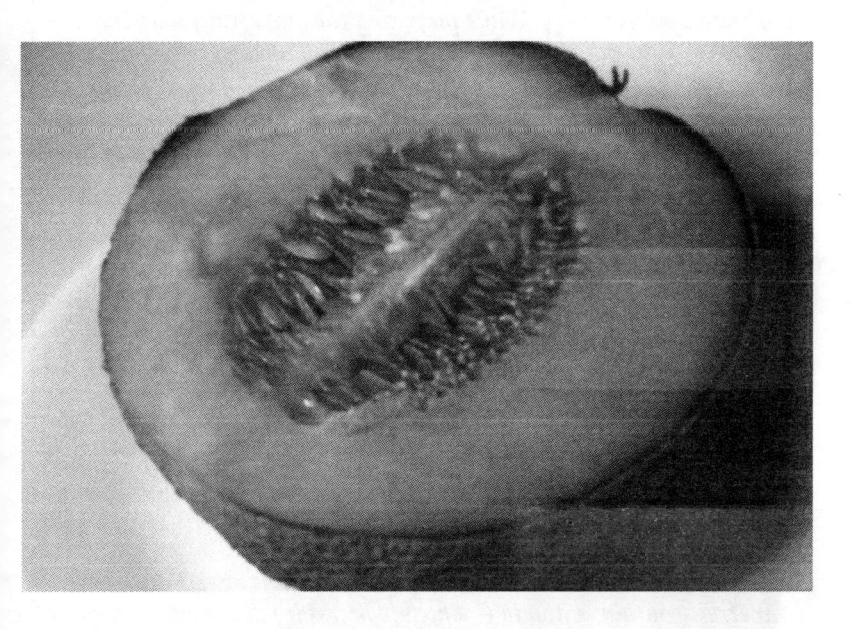

Fresh Cantaloupe (Half)

What really scares me most, more than nukes or cancer is a person without a sense of humor.

Juice for Varicose Vein

4 large fresh grapefruit	*Peel the grapefruit, leaving on as much of the outer white skin.*
4 fresh apricots	*While preparing the grapefruit, soak the apricots in a sink full of water and add 4 tablespoons of vinegar. Then wash under running water using a soft clean cloth or brush until very clean. Wash the grapefruit and cut into 4 quarters.*
	Remove the seeds from the apricots and discard. Cut into halves.
	Begin juicing starting with the grapefruit first and ending with the apricots.

Serves 2. Deliciously invigorating.

Nutritional Highlights:

Grapefruit contains vitamin C which is necessary in the maintenance of strong blood vessels. The vitamin C also stimulates the digestive tract, thereby providing regular bowel movement. Apricots contain a valuable mineral called magnesium which is vital for vascular and muscle tone. Grapefruit is also high in calcium, another important mineral for building strong bones and helps blood clotting. Grapefruit also contains bioflavonoids which are in the white pulpy part and this nutrient can strengthen the collagen structure in the vein walls.

TIPS: Avoid coffee totally as the caffeine depletes the body of oxygen. No disease can come in contact with a well-oxygenated body. Avoid wearing tight clothing and eating rubbish. Drink at least half a gallon of water on a daily basis to move the bowels and eliminate toxins. Ladies, ladies, wearing tight clothes does not guarantee you will meet a man and keep him! Do exercise, e.g. dancing, walking, stretching at least three times per week. Stay away from anything that inhibits blood circulation.

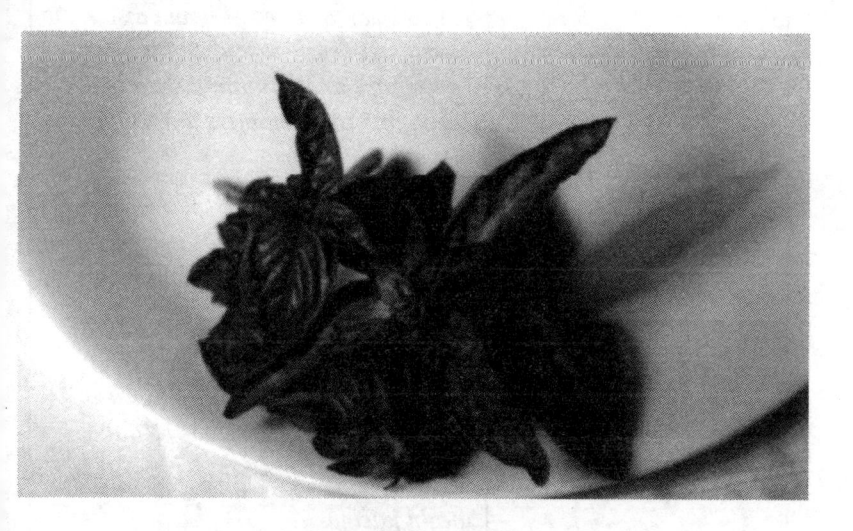

Fresh Basil Leaves

My Sister Joy's Juice for Acne Treatment

1 whole fresh cantaloupe	In a sink full of water, add 6 tablespoons of vinegar and soak the cantaloupe for 5 minutes. Drain the water.
	Add a small amount of liquid dish soap into a soft brush and scrub the cantaloupe under running water between 5 to 10 minutes until squeaky clean.
	For a final rinse, add 2 tablespoons of vinegar into a sink full of cold water and wash very well with your hands.
	Cut the cantaloupe into halves. Use a tablespoon to remove the seeds. Cut into long sections or strips. Please leave the skin/rind intact as this just about contains all the nutrients.
	Begin juicing.

Serves 2. What a delight and a world full of joy! Drink instantly.

Nutritional Highlights:

Cantaloupe contains beta carotene which stimulates the healing of wounds and burns as well as providing excellent remedy for smooth skin. Dried skin can benefit tremendously from beta carotene.

NOTES: *My baby sister, Joy, had a few acne problems when she turned 14 years old. After putting her on this diet juice for one month, her face cleared up and she regained her gorgeous looks again. But Joy also used the pulp as a facial every morning right before going to school. She* would apply the pulp on her face and let sit for 20 minutes while saying her prayers. Then after rinsing it off her face, she would apply her baby lotion. My other sister, Selin, would always tease Joy as someone who fights the mirror because Joy enjoys looking at the good result in the mirror.

Juice for Crohn's Disease

2 oz. fresh spinach ½ lb. fresh asparagus or 8 stalks	Soak the vegetables in a sink full of water, add about 4 tablespoons of vinegar or hydrogen peroxide (must be food grade). Let soak for at least 5 minutes. Then change the water and rinse for about 7 times. Place the spinach in a strainer and rinse again under running water until squeaky clean. Begin juicing starting with the asparagus first and ending with the spinach.

Serves 1. Enjoy!

Nutritional Highlights:

Spinach contains a significant amount of CoQ_{10}, an enzyme that is a naturally occurring substance which is active in the body. CoQ_{10} is also effective in reducing the rate of degenerative diseases. CoQ_{10} is also a powerful antioxidant which is necessary for defending the body from toxic free radicals by building a strong immune system. Asparagus, a member of the lily family, is a nutrient-dense low calorie food that contains more glutathione, one of the body's most potent cancer fighters - than any other food. Packed with folic acid, which has been shown to help prevent birth defects, asparagus is treasured for its ability to nourish and strengthen blood vessels.

TIPS: Chron's disease is a very serious illness. It is an ulceration of the colon and one can lose blood, weight, and nutrients. Therefore, the best way to keep this disease away is to keep the colon extremely clean.

Juice for High Fever

1 oz. fresh thyme 6 stalks of celery 4 large carrots	Peel off the skin of the carrots and cut the leaves at the stem to get rid of the pesticides.
	Place both the carrots and celery into a sink full of water and add 2 tablespoons of vinegar. Let soak for 3 minutes.
	Under running water using a scouring brush, scrub the celery and the carrots very clean.
	Place the thyme in either a strainer or a small plate and rinse very well.
	Begin juicing starting with the celery, then the thyme, then the carrots, and ending with the celery.

Serves 2. Enjoy! Cool and refreshing.

Nutritional Highlights:

Celery contains organic sodium which maintains proper blood pressure and provides us the primary support for our blood pressure. Thyme is an herb that contains vitamin C and it is well known for its powerful antioxidants and helps protect against environmental damage. Carrots contain potassium which is an essential mineral that may help lower cholesterol deposits in the blood stream. A combination of both potassium

Juicing For Your Soul

and sodium helps to regulate the heart beat and balance fluids. TIPS: Take a cool shower to lower the body temperature. Try eating about 6 oz. of food until the fever drops. Drink at least half a gallon of distilled water to compensate for the loss that occurs with fever. Potassium and sodium is lost when fluid is lost, hence the replacement is vital.

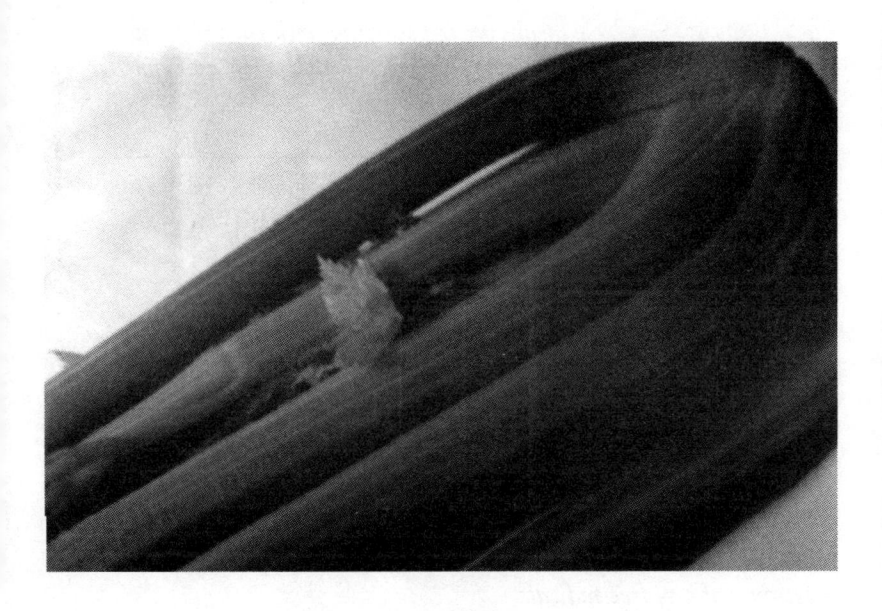

Celery Stalks

Prevention is better than cure.

Juice for Prostate Cancer

2 qts. fresh cranberries	Place the cranberries in a strainer and add 3 tablespoons of vinegar. Rinse extremely well under running water for at least 5 minutes.
6 fresh tangerines	
4 cloves fresh garlic	Peel off the skins of both the tangerines and the garlic and wash until clean. Cut the tangerines into 4 quarters each. Do not remove the rinds—the white stringy pulpy part.
	Begin juicing starting with the tangerines, then the berries, then the garlic, and ending with the tangerines.

Serves 2. Uuuuuummmmmmm!

Nutritional Highlights:

Cranberries contain quininic acid which is capable of removing any toxins from the kidneys and testicles. This is an excellent juice for preventing cancer of the testicles. Garlic is such a simple life-saving remedy. It can stop a host of disease-causing viruses. It strengthens the immune system and has natural antibiotic and anticancer properties. Tangerines are part of the citrus fruits and contain a very significant amount of the A vitamin, an essential nutrient for healing the urinary tract and a destroyer of any free radicals.

FYI: Please talk to your doctor before starting on this juice.

My father once said to me, "One has to have grace about life, see it as a noble pursuit of the days try to embrace it as opposing to living through it."

Juicing For Your Soul

Juice for Cervical Cancer

1/4 lb. fresh kale 1 lb. fresh large red tomatoes	Soak the vegetables in a biodegradable soap for 2 minutes to remove any and all of the chemical residues. Wet a clean washcloth, add 2 tablespoons of vinegar and scrub tomatoes under running water until squeaky clean. Place the kale in a strainer and rinse thoroughly using your hand. Cut off the black tip on top of the tomatoes and cut into 4 sections each. Start juicing adding the tomatoes into the hopper first, followed by the kale, and ending with the tomatoes.

Serves 1. Enjoy!

Nutritional Highlights:

Both kale and tomatoes are rich in a substance called phytochemicals, an extremely powerful antioxidant that is necessary for blocking the processes that lead to cancer. These phytochemicals can help remove the molecules that attack healthy cells in the body. They are a powerful immune protector and help the body to excrete toxins. Tomatoes and Kale also nourishes and supports the immune system by preserving oxygen in the body.

My parents once told me, "You must radiate exuberance,"

Juice for Bruises

1 whole fresh unripe pineapple 12 oz. fresh raspberries	Soak the pineapple in water and add in 2 tablespoons of liquid detergent. Allow to soak for 2 minutes. Using a hard vegetable brush, scrub the pineapple under running water for at least 2 minutes. Add 4 tablespoons of vinegar and wash very well again until thoroughly clean. Cut off the stems at both ends. Cut the pineapple in half and cut into strips. Soak the raspberries in a bowl of water with 2 tablespoons of vinegar and rinse well. Begin juicing starting with the pineapple first and ending with the berries.

Serves 2.
Deliciously satisfying!!! This one is irresistible! Smelling like a fresh pineapple, you'll feel good all day after a sip.

Nutritional Highlights:

Pineapples contain vitamin C, an essential element necessary for protecting the skin tissues as well as providing oxygen to any injured cells. Pineapples also contain the vitamin B-complex which is another vital element in healing any skin problem. Raspberries contain some valuable nutrients—one being an antioxidant. It is an excellent aid against free radical damage to the body. The B-complex vitamin increases energy and combats stress.

Juice to Help Prevent Measles in Children

12 tangerines, large ones 4 cloves fresh garlic,	Peel the tangerines and the garlic. Leave on as much as the pulpy white part/strings of the tangerines as you can. You can actually use your fingers to remove the outer yellow skin part of the tangerine. Wash thoroughly under running water. You may add a tablespoon of vinegar and rinse off with water until squeaky clean. Cut the tangerines in half, crosswise. Begin juicing starting with the tangerines first and ending with the garlic.

Serves 2. Enjoy!

Nutritional Highlights:

Tangerines contain a substantial amount of vitamin A, an essential vitamin that decreases the severity of measles in children. It offers a host of benefits including protection against viral disease. One of the symptoms of measles is inflammation of the eyes; therefore, the vitamin A is important for the health tissue of the eye. Garlic contains rich nutrients that can treat any disease. Garlic will cure various ailments of the eyes and the skin.

TIPS: *Please stay away from other people to avoid spreading the disease. Drink lots of good water. Good hygiene is crucial at all times, especially at this point of the disease by taking a shower three times daily!!*

Juice For Cataracts

12 oz. blueberries, fresh please 1 whole unripe fresh pineapple 3 cloves fresh garlic	Soak the berries in a bowl full of water. Add 3 tablespoons of vinegar. Let soak for 2 minutes. In the meantime, soak the pineapple in sink full of water with the additional of 3 tablespoons of vinegar. You may add a bit of dishwashing soap and scrub thoroughly under fast running water until all the dirt is gone. Rinse thoroughly. Rinse the berries very well in a strainer under running water. Wash the garlic thoroughly as well. Cut off the pineapple ends and discard. Cut the pineapple into strips and start juicing beginning with the pineapples first, then the berries, then the garlic, and ending with the pineapples.

Serves 3. What a delight!!!

Nutritional Highlights:
Blueberries are packed with nutrient-rich elements that will tone and strengthen the uterine wall. Blueberries also contain antioxidants which

will prevent cataracts and macular degeneration. Pineapples contain the mineral called potassium which is an important factor in maintaining the muscle and nerve systems. The benefits of garlic are too numerous to list. Garlic contains many properties that will eliminate any disease from the body. They have a wide range of beneficial effects on the circulatory and central nervous systems.

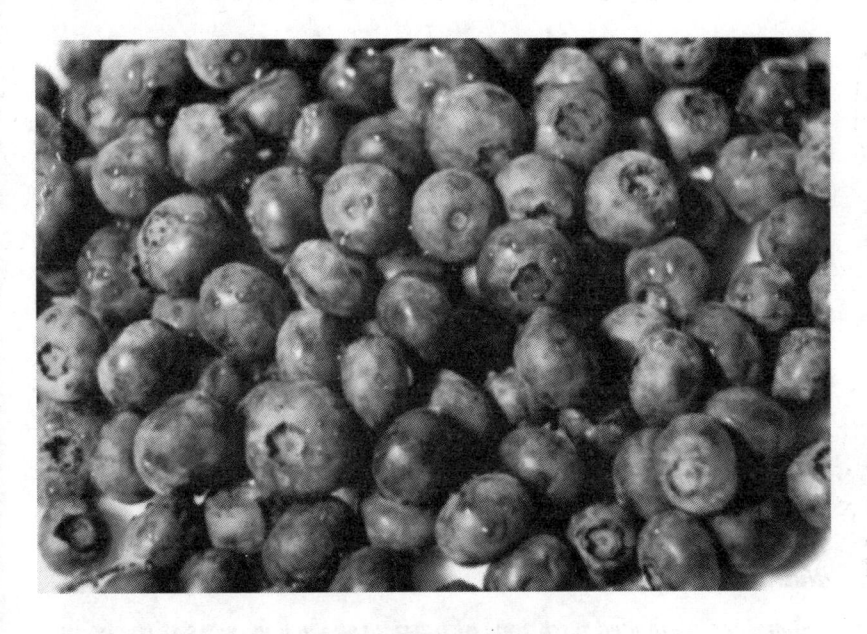

Fresh Blueberries

"My one wish for the world is unity"

Juice for Muscle Mass

4 medium size apples 8 tangerines 3 cloves of fresh garlic	Soak the apples in a biodegradable soap for 2 minutes. Scrub thoroughly clean under running water; or better yet, peel off the skin of the apples. This will remove all the chemical residues. Core the apples and cut into quarters. Peel the tangerines and discard the skin. Peel the garlic and discard the skin as well. Wash all ingredients thoroughly. Begin juicing starting with an apple, then the garlic, followed by the tangerines, and finally the apples again.

Serves 3. Enjoy. Tastes delicious!!!

Nutritional Highlights:

Tangerines are loaded with tons of nutrients which may assist the body in the maintenance of rebuilding existing tissue. Vitamin C may also help the body heal itself by eliminating toxins. The C vitamin also promotes the production of anti stress hormones by breaking down the free radicals. Apples contain calcium, an important mineral that will help increase a person's peak bone mass. Calcium is also important in maintaining healthy hearts, skin, strong muscles and nerves. Garlic is a natural herb that contains all the nutrients that will increase energy and vitality, as well as relieve stress levels.

Juice to Relieve Hiccups

2 large cucumbers 1/4 lb. fresh ginger root 1 whole fresh lemon	Using a produce brush, scrub the ginger root and lemon under running water, adding some vinegar and rinse thoroughly. Soak the cucumbers in water and add 3 tablespoons of vinegar. Let sit for 3 minutes. Using either a clean white washcloth or a brush, scrub very well under running water until it feels squeaky clean. Dice the ginger root, cut the lemon into 4 sections, and cut the cucumber in half, crosswise. Begin juicing starting with a cucumber, then the lemon and the ginger root, and ending with the cucumbers.

Serves 1. Unbelievable relief. WOW!!

Nutritional Highlights:

Cucumbers contain rich nutrients that have a calming effect on the body. Cucumbers contain magnesium, an important mineral for maintaining our physiological functions as well as preserving the vigor of the heart and brain. Ginger roots contain sodium, a primarily needed mineral in strengthening skeletal structures and essential for proper body functioning and overall good health. Lemons contain some iron which enhances resistance to infections. The iron in lemons also support mental abilities and provide a sense of general well-being.

TIPS: *Eating slowly and proper relaxation after eating could help eliminate the hiccups. You may drink this juice 20 minutes before meals to sooth your lungs.*

Juice for Depression

6 oz. raspberries 1 whole fresh unripe pineapple 2 oz. fresh thyme leaves	Place the raspberries in a strainer and add 2 tablespoons of vinegar. Rinse thoroughly and set aside. Place the thyme in a strainer and add a tablespoon of vinegar. Rinse thoroughly as well and set aside. Soak the pineapple in a biodegradable liquid washer for 2 minutes or longer. Scrub thoroughly under running water until squeaky clean. As a final rinse, place the pineapple into a bowl of water. Add 2 tablespoons of vinegar and rinse well. Cut off both ends and discard. Cut the pineapple into small pieces, enough to fit into the pulper. Begin juicing starting with the pineapple, then the berries, then the thyme, and ending with the pineapple.

Serves 3. Enjoy!!!

Nutritional Highlights:

Raspberries have a high content of magnesium, a mineral that is quite beneficial in reducing both depression and migraine headaches. Thyme contains calcium which will supply the nervous system with some serenity. Thyme will also help eliminate toxins and parasites from the body. Pineapples contain folic acid which provides important tools for normal functioning of the brain.

TIPS: *Always think positive. Surround yourself with happy people at all times. You must invent your own happiness. Do not do things that you will later regret in life; that is, let your conscious be your protection. Do right and pray at least morning and night.*

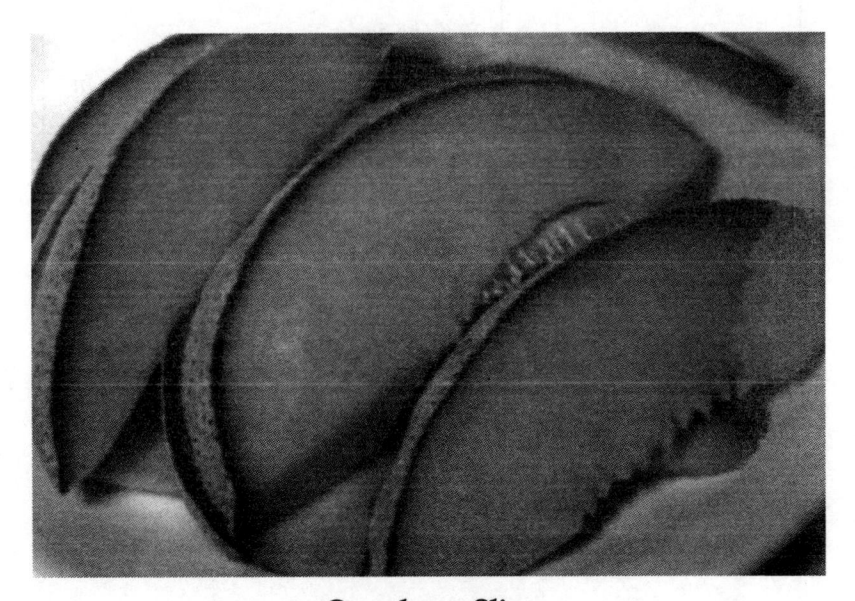

Cantaloupe Slices

My parents said to me, "You must get to really know a couple of people who are poor. The world looks very different when you're down and out. Look around, you'll find an opportunity to have a conversation with a person who is poor. Do so."

Juice to Relieve Arteriosclerosis

3 large grapefruits 11 oz. fresh blueberries 3 cloves fresh garlic	Peel the grapefruits leaving on as much of the white membrane parts as possible. Wash the grapefruits and cut into small sections. Peel the garlic. Place both the garlic and the berries in a strainer. Add 2 tablespoons of vinegar and rinse very well under running water. Proceed juicing starting with the grapefruit first, then the berries, then the garlic, and ending with the grapefruits.

Serves 2. Have fun and be well!!!

Nutritional Highlights:

Grapefruits contain vitamin C, a potent antioxidant which will increase circulation to the extremities and support the body's immune system in its resistance to heart disease. Blueberries contain vitamin A, a powerful element that will destroy free radicals as well as to protect the mucous membranes of the lungs. Garlic contains essential nutrients that will regulate the heart, enhance immunity, and inhibit any fatty deposits in the arteries. Thiamine can also be found in garlic, an important vitamin for maintaining the heart.

Eat your food the way nature intended—fresh.

Juicing For Your Soul

Juice to Relieve Candidiasis

1/4 lb. fresh red onion (remove outer skin) 6 oz. fresh blackberries 6 tangerines	In a bowl full of water, add 3 tablespoons of vinegar, the onions, and the blackberries. Let soak for 2 minutes. Place them in a strainer and rinse very well. Peel the tangerines and discard the skin and wash thoroughly. Cut the tangerines into 12 segments and slice the onions into small sections. Begin juicing starting with the tangerines first, then the onions, and the berries, and ending with the tangerines.

Serves 1. What a life's delight!!!

Nutritional Highlights:

Onions contain quercitin, a vitamin-like nutrient that has a valuable antiallergen which can slow down the production of other allergy-related diseases. Onions have the key nutrients to remove toxins from the body. Blackberries are rich in vitamin C which can help rid the body of worms and any other internal parasites. Tangerines contain magnesium, a mineral necessary for soothing the nerves and it can relieve any aches.

Manners and civility count for everything.

Juicing For Your Soul

Juice for Colitis

1 oz. fresh marjoram leaves	Peel the tangerines and discard the skins.
12 oz. large ripe fresh mangoes	Soak both the berries and the mangoes in a biodegradable soap with water to remove any chemical residue. Wash all ingredients thoroughly until quite clean.
8 tangerines	
	Cut the mangoes into pieces and remove the large pits.
	Cut the tangerines into halves.
	Begin juicing starting with some of the tangerines first, then the mangoes, the berries, the marjoram leaves, and ending with the tangerines.

Serves 2. Delightfully inviting!!!

Nutritional Highlights:

Blackberries contain magnesium, an element that will provide an overall sense of well-being. Mangoes are very high in fiber, important for eliminating rubbish out of the system. Fiber will also provide a regular bowel movement. The likelihood of any ailment to occur in the body will be low if the bowels are emptied on a regular basis. Marjoram is an herb that contains exceptional nutrients which will inhibit growth sores and it is also helpful for the digestive system. Tangerines are full of phosphorus, a mineral necessary for a healthy nervous system.

TIPS: When one is plagued with colitis, one of the symptoms is constant loss of water though the lower digestive tract which could result in dehydration. Therefore, it is essential to drink the above recommended juice at least three times per day along with ten glasses of distilled water.

Juice for Bursitis

7 stalks celery 2 oz. fresh tarragon 3 large carrots	Under running water, scrub the celery one by one using a soft brush until thoroughly cleansed. Place the tarragon in a strainer. Add a few drops of vinegar and rinse well. Scrape off the skin of the carrots. Cut off both ends and discard, and then rinse well. Cut the carrots. Begin juicing adding the celery first, then the tarragon, then the carrots, and ending with the celery.

Serves 3. Enjoy!!!

Nutritional Highlights:

Tarragon is an herb which can help curb pains or swellings. The B complex vitamins also provide quick energy. Carrots are full of carotenes which are powerful antioxidants that will provide a strong immunity against any disease. The carotene acts as a defender to the whole body system. Celery is also full of the vitamin B-complex—an indispensable substance needed by the body for tissue maintenance.

TIPS: A 10-minute daily stretching should help. Learn to manage stress by not getting hyped up over little things.

Juice for Canker Sores

8 tangerines	Peel off the skin of the tangerines and discard.
2 nectarines	
1 lb. Golden Globe grapes (with seeds)	Soak the nectarines, grapes, and berries in a biodegradable liquid and wash for 2 minutes.
5-8 oz. fresh blackberries	Rinse thoroughly, adding 2 tablespoons of vinegar.
	Use a soft washcloth or brush and scrub the nectarines to rid them of any chemical spray.
	Cut the tangerines in halves. Cut the nectarines, remove the pits, and discard.
	Begin juicing starting with the tangerines, then the berries, grapes, nectarines, and ending with the tangerines.

Serves 3. One of my favorites. Enjoy!

Nutritional Highlights:

Tangerines have adequate amounts of the vitamin B-complex which will help in the general condition of one's well-being. Nectarines contain a significant amount of vitamin A which will provide healing to the mucous membranes of the lips. The seeds in the grapes contain pycnogenol which is an antioxidant that may prevent any sores from forming. Blackberries contain folic acid, an essential element for reproduction of all body cells.

Juicing For Your Soul

TIPS: *Add a small teaspoon of vinegar to your toothpaste before brushing. Overall proper hygiene is extremely important. Eat no spicy foods.*

Juice to Halt Cravings

5 oz. blueberries *1 whole fresh green pineapple* *1 qt. fresh strawberries*	*Soak the berries in a bowl full of cold water.* *Add 2 tablespoons of vinegar and rinse well.* *Soak the pineapple in a biodegradable liquid wash.* *Under running water, scrub the pineapple very hard for at least 10 minutes until very clean.* *Cut the pineapple into small pieces.* *Start juicing beginning with the pineapple, then the blueberries, the stberries, and ending with the pineapple.*

Serves 2. Enjoy!

Note: *You must juice the pineapple with the skin to get the nutritional value.*

Nutritional Highlights:

Both the blueberries, stberries, and the pineapple all contain an element called inositol which reduces both sugar and carbohydrate cravings. Inositol also possesses antidepressant qualities that tell the brain you are not hungry.

NOTE: *Do not skip meals as it will only intensify food cravings.*

Juice to Help Urinary Infection

3 cloves garlic 3 fresh pears 2 mangoes	Peel off the skin of the garlic and wash thoroughly. Soak both the mangoes and pears in a sink full of water. Add 2 tablespoons of vinegar. Let soak for 2 minutes. Scrub with a soft brush or a clean white washcloth until thoroughly clean. Cut the pears and remove the seeds. Cut the mangoes and remove the pits inside. Cut both the mangoes and pears into small pieces. Proceed juicing beginning with the pears, then the garlic, the mangoes, and ending with the pears.

Serves 1.
Enjoy! Consume immediately to get the full medicinal value.

Nutritional Highlights:

Garlic contains high amounts of zinc, a mineral which has an effect on inhibiting fungus and strengthens the immune system. Garlic also has antiseptic and diuretic properties. Both mangoes and pears are very high in fiber, a physiological necessity that has a stimulating effect on digestion and reduces the formation of gas. In addition, fiber will help rid your body of toxic pollutants.

My parents once said to me, "Give thanks to people who deserve it. Develop an attitude of gratitude. Cultivate the habit of looking for opportunities to thank others. You won't have to look far."

Juice for Teething Infants

| 10 tangerines
1 qt. strawberries
(fresh, please) | Peel off the skin of the tangerines and wash very well until clean.

Remove the stems of the strawberries and soak in a sink full of water with 3 tablespoons of vinegar. Let soak for a few minutes.

Pour the strawberries into a strainer and rinse several times under running water.

Cut the tangerines into small sections.

Proceed juicing starting with the tangerines and ending with the strawberries. |

Serves 1.
Gratifying and delightful tasting. Enjoy!

Nutritional Highlights:

Tangerines are full of vitamin C which is vital to collagen formation, the connective substance in all cells. The more stress you experience, the more the need for this vitamin is highly recommended. Strawberries are highly concentrated in leucine, an essential amino acid that helps protect muscle. Leucine will also help promote the healing of skin and muscle tissue. It lowers elevated blood sugar levels. Besides the strawberries containing this essential amino acid, it also contains zinc, a mineral for aiding enzymes in the digestion process.

Charity begins at home and it should never end there."

Juice for Prostate Enlargement

1 lb. kohlrabi root 1/4 lb. fresh parsley 2 oz. fresh ginger root	Scrape off the skin of the kohlrabi root if desired and wash thoroughly under running water. Soak the parsley and ginger root in a sink full of water. Add 2 tablespoons of vinegar and let soak for 3 minutes. Pour the parsley into a strainer and rinse well until very clean. Use a brush and scrub the ginger root under running water until all the traces of dirt have disappeared. Cut the kohlrabi roots and the ginger root into small pieces. Begin juicing starting with the kohlrabi, then the parsley leaves, then the ginger root, and ending with the kohlrabi roots.

Serves 1.
Enjoy! This drink bears within it an extraordinary secret of vitality!!!

Nutritional Highlights:

Ginger roots are high in zinc, a mineral that contains all the essential nutrients for normal prostate function. It will help ease inflammation by reducing the discomfort of urination. Both the kohlrabi root and parsley contain vitamin C which is an amazing vitamin for detoxifying the body *and can be very effective in treating prostate disease. Kohlrabi root does quite a remarkable job in controlling inflammation.*

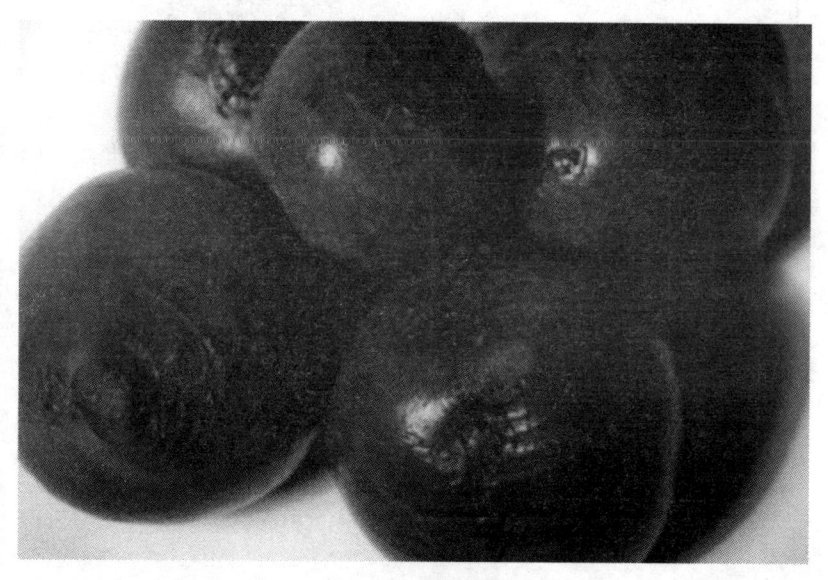

Beets (Whole)

Help a refugee. There are millions of men, women, and children with no homes. No one of us can help them all, but each of us can and must do something.

Juice for an Infant's Well-Being

1 whole watermelon	*Soak the whole watermelon in a biodegradable liquid wash in a sink full of water. Let soak for 2 minutes.* *Use a clean wash cloth or brush and thoroughly scrub under fast running water until very clean. You may add some vinegar and rinse under water again. Cut the watermelon into quarters first and then into smaller pieces to fit into the pulper.* *Simply begin juicing everything including the skin, rinds, and seeds.*

Serves 6.
Mouth-watering delight!!!

Nutritional Highlights:

Watermelon contains a remarkable valuable nutrient. It contains an essential amino acid called isoleucine which may help to assist optimal growth in infants and may play a role, early on, in preventing certain retardation. Watermelon is a powerful antianxiety food. It is excellent for the brain as a transmitter for nerve cells. I would rather call it a health-giving substance. The vitamin C content in the watermelon will help build resistance to infections by protecting children's immunity.

Here's an invitation to a fine life!

Juice to Relieve Lupus

4 kiwis 3 cups fresh cranberries 6 oranges	Peel the kiwis and oranges leaving on as much as the white membrane as possible. Add 2 tablespoons of vinegar. Wash the kiwis and oranges. Then cut into halves. Begin juicing starting with the oranges first, the kiwis second, the cranberries third, and ending with the oranges.

Serves 3. Enjoy yourselves!

Nutritional Highlights:

Cranberries contain some nutritional substances that will acidify the urine and at the same time destroy bacteria build-up and promote healing of the bladder. Cranberries also contain magnesium that will fight chronic fatigue syndrome. Oranges are rich in calcium, a mineral that will strengthen bone. Calcium is also important for regulating muscular tone and transmitting nerve impulses throughout the body and the brain. Kiwis are full of vitamin C, an essential vitamin for healing sores and as an immune system enhancer. The vitamin C will also reduce inflammation.

"Hate destroys the vessel that it is carried in"

Juice to Ease Rheumatoid Arthritis

1 whole fresh pineapple 4 nectarines Note: You must juice the pineapple with the skin intact.	Soak the ingredients in water and add 2 tablespoons vinegar. Let soak for 2 minutes. Using a soft brush under running water, scrub all the ingredients until squeaky clean, up to the point that no traces of filth/dirt can be found. Remove any stem from the pineapple. Cut the pineapple into small pieces. Cut the nectarines into halves and remove the pits. Begin juicing starting with the half of the pineapple first, then the nectarines, and then the rest of the pineapple.

Serves 3. Quite a delight. Hope you enjoy!

Nutritional Highlights:

Pineapple contains the vitamin B complex which is necessary for energy production. Pineapple contains other essential nutrients that are necessary for bone growth as well as in preventing further damage to joints. Nectarines are rich in essential nutrients such as potassium and calcium and are both crucial for building strong bones that are needed for muscle growth. These minerals may also help prevent bone loss associated with arthritis.

"Life is a celebration of love and generosity," my parents said to me.

Juice for Itchy/Swollen Eye

4 pears, preferably large ones 6 tangerines 1 oz. fresh chives	Peel the tangerines, preferably using your fingers to pull off the skin. Soak the pears in vinegar and water for 2 minutes. Using a soft cloth, scrub them and rinse well under running water. Place the chives in a strainer and using your fingers, wash well under running water until clean. Cut the tangerines into segments. Cut the pears and remove the seeds. Begin juicing starting with some of the pears, then the chives, then the tangerines, and ending with the rest of the pears.

Serves 2. What a powerhouse of natural goodness!!!

Nutritional Highlights:

Pears are rich in vitamin C which is necessary for strengthening the mucous membranes and helps clean the internal organs. The vitamin C has a potent effect upon the lymphatic system and related glands. Tangerines are high in folic acid, an important element for healthy cells. Folic acid can also help prevent stunted growth in children. Tangerines also contain phosphorous, a mineral that is essential in treating relief of muscle cramps and nervous exhaustion. Chives will improve the body's overall health and fend off illnesses.

TIPS: Be sure to get a good night's sleep.

Juice for Scurvy/Dry Lips

4 kiwis 5 oz. blackberries 6 tangerines	Peel off the skin of both the kiwis and the tangerines. Wash thoroughly clean. Place the blackberries in a strainer. Add 2 tablespoons of vinegar and wash until very clean. Cut the tangerines into segments, the kiwis into halves. Begin juicing starting with the tangerines first, then the kiwis, berries, and ending with the tangerines again.

Serves 2. Have a great feeling!!!

Nutritional Highlights:

All the above fruits are full of vitamin C which helps prevent scurvy. Vitamin C is a powerful antioxidant that will destroy free radical scavengers and will also destroy harmful elements. The C vitamin is useful for tissue growth and repair, and it will also eliminate colds and influenza. Blackberries are such a powerful antioxidant that its other benefits are often overlooked. Decreased inflammation, improvement in circulation and vision, and skin protection are just a few of the possible benefits.

Jealousy is a sign of insecurity which is a key to disease.

Juice for Dry Hair

2 lbs. endive 1/4 lb. fresh ginger root 1 lb. carrots	Thoroughly wash the endive under fast running water. You may add a few drops of vinegar to get rid of chemicals and pesticides.
	Scrub the ginger root with a soft vegetable brush and rinse well. Peel off the skin of the carrots. Cut off both ends and scrub thoroughly until all traces of dirt are removed.
	Dice the ginger and cut the carrots so as to fit into the juice hopper.
	Begin juicing starting with the endive, then the ginger, and ending with the carrots.

Serves 3. Great tasting!!!

Nutritional Highlights:

Both the endive and carrots are high in niacin and vitamin A which are important for eliminating stress. These nutrients are also excellent for the appearance of vibrant skin and renewal of cells. Ginger root is an excellent source of many vitamins and minerals necessary for antiaging.

Note: Dry hair can result from stress and vitamin deficiency. It may be necessary to drink this juice on a regular basis until the situation is corrected.

> *"There's nothing more fabulous than having spiritual credentials"*

Selin's (my sister) Summer Cleansing Juice

3 lbs. fresh chives 2 lbs. apples	Soak chives in cold water. Add 2 teaspoons of vinegar. Let sit for a few minutes, while peeling the skin off of the apples. Wash both the apples and the chives thoroughly clean. Begin juicing starting with the apples and ending with the chives.

Serves 2. Delightfully refreshing!!!

Nutritional Highlights:

Chives are really nutritious. They contain rich nutrients that can supercharge the immune system. Chives contain fiber, nourishment for preventing constipation. Apples also contain fiber which can boost your energy level and maximize your body's healing power. The vitamins and mineral contents in apples can also be used in enhancing liver function.

A house is not a home unless it contains good food for the mind, body, and soul.

Anna Omenka's (my 119 year old great, great grandmother) Secrets to Joy, the Good Life, and Longevity

- First and foremost, we should all exist as human beings and not as a race.
- We should define our happiness & sense of purpose in life by helping others.
- We all belong to each other.
- We must radiate life at all times.
- We must keep things simple.
- We must not overeat to avoid stress.
- We must not engage in war because it is a violation of human rights.
- We all have a right to live in peace as it contributes to a lengthy life span.
- We must respect food if we want respect for our body.
- We must not be judgmental; there is validity in everybody's story.
- Always respect others; it is a very high spiritual value.
- We have to cultivate our own happiness.
- We must live a happy life, doing the most with what we have, with delight.

Nourishment elements such as love, humor, passion, forgiveness, wonder, sharing, giving, hope, enthusiasm, compassion, and joy stimulate the immune system. They help our bodies fight infection and stimulate natural killer cells that fight disease and affect the general way we care for ourselves and others. Conversely, when anger, resentment, hate, envy, ego, ambivalence, prejudice,

Juicing For Your Soul

guilt, boredom, loneliness, and fear are held for any length of time, they will suppress our natural protective systems and make us feel worse.

Living a happy, positive, vibrant life is crucial for our overall well-being. Offering the same friendly personality and sharing to the world at large will make it a better place for all.

And, finally, you must have love in your heart as it can enliven our whole life.

My great, great grandma, at 119 years old, is still healthy and fit. Yes, she still has the strength to take her 30-minute walk and does her gardening daily without fail. She still has all her faculties together, meaning her eyes, ears, taste, senses, smell, uses no cane for walking, no hunchback, and has all her teeth.

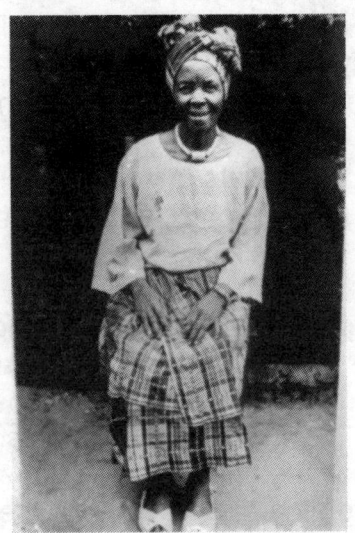

Anna Omenka, my great, great Grandmother

Juicing For Your Soul

Anna Omenka's Secret Juice for Joy and Longevity

4 lbs. fresh ugu leaves	Wash ugu leaves thoroughly under fast running water for at least 7 minutes until no traces of dirt can be found.
	Using your hand, grab a bunch of ugu leaves and place under the hopper, pushing though and begin juicing.

Serves 2. Drink immediately for full nourishment.

Nutritional Highlights:

Ugu leaves contain many important nutrients such as folic acid which guard against chronic fatigue and preserves our genetic integrity. Ugu also contains many powerful antioxidants, a necessity for the heart to pump strongly and efficiently. The antioxidants in the ugu leaves also will: a) boost both physical and cellular energy; b) strengthen the immune system; c) normalize blood pressure and cholesterol; d) slow down the aging process; e) promote healthy arteries and circulation; f) detoxify and nurture our liver, kidneys, and other organs by eliminating toxins from our body.

Note: *If ugu leaves are not available, substitute fresh kale.*

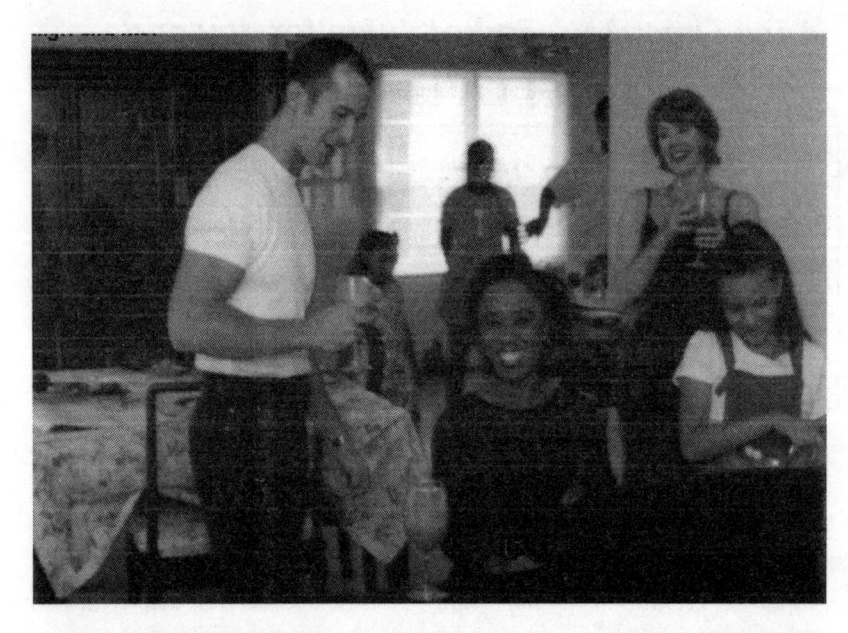

Above: Phiner sharing a great time at home with friends while playing the piano. From left: Actor Steve Baird, Phiner Dike (myself), Actress/Model Kim Hendrickson, and Terry, granddaughter of Cleveland Cavalier General Manager

Juicing For Your Soul

What Others Are Saying About Phiner Dike

"Phiner Dike has made a huge impact on my life. She has the unique ability to make people feel great. Phiner Dike exudes energy and enthusiasm. She knows how to live the great life. She is an inspiration. My life has been touched by a very special person."

— Melanie Biel

"What Phiner has to offer is priceless. I use her book everyday on juicing and I will continue to do so as long as I am alive."

— David Griffen

"Phiner Dike has taught me patience, trust, and relaxation as they relate to health, art, and life in general. She certainly has the secrets for living the good life. The closest I feel I have to come to genius has been with Phiner Dike."

— Christopher

"Phiner is a fine and remarkable human being."

— Lorna Davis, M.D.

"To change our weight we must change our diet. Phiner Dike's books show how."

— John Cox

"The most dedicated and reliable human being I've ever met."

— *Bill Morley*

"As proud as a peacock."

— *Carl Gordon, Actor*

"Sensitive and compassionate."

— *Dr. Tillman Bauknight*

"Fortunately, I met Phiner Dike at a time when I was experiencing bouts of ongoing leg and ankle swelling problems. During that first meeting, I found her personable and concerned enough to confide to her the discomfort and stress these health problems were causing me. Immediately, she introduced me to a simplistic and natural approach to alleviate these problems with a beneficial by-product—adopting a healthier lifestyle. As a result of that conversation, I purchased Phiner's book. It combines information on the extraordinary dynamics of certain foods' catalystic healing properties to the body while introducing an easy and delicious way to enjoy the benefits of these foods. She is able to provide surprising food combinations enhanced by the aid of a juicer which are amazingly tasteful. Since reading Phiner's book, I have a new kitchen staple—a juicer. I also know which foods are "user friendly" and which are not."

— *Joan*

"Distinctive and thoroughly lovable."

— *David Stuart*

"With malice toward none, with charity for all."

— *Sade, Singer*

"Very effeminate in nature."

— *Akumoah Family*

"Elegance at every turn."

— *James Earl Jones, Actor*

"As intelligent as she is beautiful."

— *Robert B. Young*
Assistant VP, Society Corp.

"Phiner has an incredible energy and passion for the good life. She lives life with a great intensity only few can equal."

— *Annette Stanley, Computer Progammer*

"My skin looks so much healthier. My acne has cleared up. My skin is better and so is my self-esteem with Phiner's juicing."

- Kim, Actress/Model

"I look younger, I have had no more cold sores on my lips, and I can feel the effects of Phiner's juices! Phiner, keep up the good work!"

- Richard Vargo, Professor of Law

"Effervescently refreshing to the taste buds...leaving you with a sense of having just ingested renewal nectar!"

- Robin Carolan, M.D.

"I was first impressed by Phiner's sparkling personality and her beauty. Her pride in her heritage is evident, as is the generous spirit she demonstrates to reach out to kids in trouble. Of course, we all flipped for her cooking! Phiner is a culinary genius. The foods she taught us to prepare were delicious, and she was a patient and detailed instructor."

- Martha Shaw, Youth Worker
Safespace Teen Shelter/Teen Outreach

"Extraordinary talented lady who inspires and stirs your senses."

- Frank Lazar, Stockbroker

Juicing For Your Soul

"Phiner Dike introduced me to one of her juice concoctions. While I was skeptical of drinking this green stuff, I know that she would never recommend anything that was not completely healthy. Here goes—down the hatch. Surprise, surprise!! The cantaloupe juice, while an ugly color, due to the chlorophyll in the rind, was pleasantly refreshing. It was light, slightly sweet, and delightfully flavorful."

- James E. Fieldler

"Phiner Dike is a very physically fit woman. I gave her a massage of her skin and it is so firm and tight that I could hardly pinch or roll it."

- Jack Fraas, Massotherapist

"Phiner got me excited about juicing, especially since I've gone vegan a few years ago. A couple of times per week I use her recipes just for general well-being and energy because they work. Even when I have leftover fruits and vegetables that don't quite make up one of her recipes, I'll put them in the juicer anyway and drink it, not necessarily always the best tasting "surprise" concoction, but I know it is giving me a powerful vitamin and mineral punch."

- Doris Lee

"If the world had a royal family of health, she would be a princess."

- Robert Delmontique, Author

"Success wouldn't spoil Phiner, my daughter. It's going to give her permission to do so much more for the world. She'll be able to be totally outrageous and have people donate airplanes to bring humanity together. She's a social change artist. She's a role model. She wants to show the world it's possible that instead of worshiping money and power, hate and prejudice, to worship compassion and generosity, fun and love."

- Mr. C. Dike, Phinner Dike's father
Architectural Engineer

"I see a person of rare beauty. Phiner illuminates the paths of all who encounter her."

- Christopher Richards, M.D.

"No one who ever met her didn't feel that life was much better that minute."

- Mary Adom, Model

"She was delicately reared and accustomed to the refinements of life."

- Helen Oto, Model

"Phiner is—and I do not say this lightly—World's healthiest."

- Verle Setrick, Model

Juicing For Your Soul

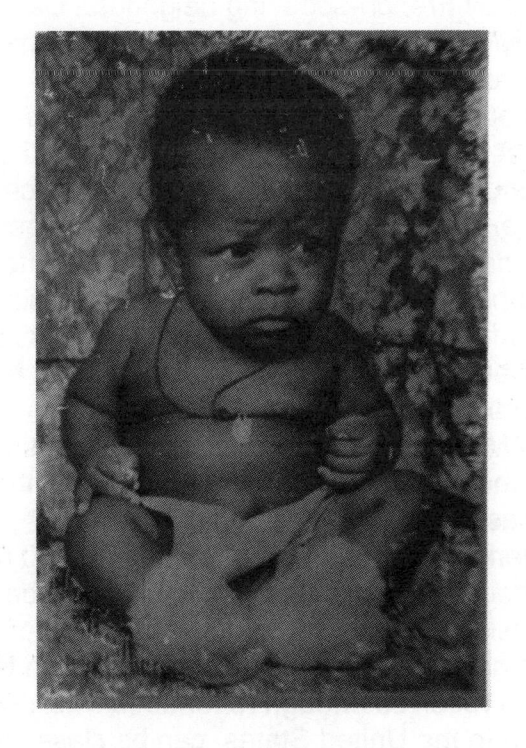

Baby photo of Phiner Dike

A Brief Background of Nigeria

On October 1, 1960, Nigeria became independent. Prior to that, it was a British colony. It is about 356,000 square miles in area and lies within the tropics. It is a nation in which English is the official language. Nigeria is surrounded by French-speaking neighbors, Dahomey on the West, Niger to the North, Chad to the Northeast, and Cameroon to the East.

Although English is the official language of government, education, and the mass media, there are 200 indigenous languages and dialects. As such, in the city slums and rural villages, better English is seldom used. Nigeria is inhabited by more than 200 different ethnic groups. The main language in the Northern area is Hausa, of which about 20 million people speak. Other languages are: Ibo—spoken in the Southeast; and Yoruba–spoken in the Southwest. The northern people are mostly Muslim, whereas Christianity has its greatest impact on the people in the south, particularly the Ibos and Yorubas.

Nigeria in inhabited by an estimated 100 million people. About half the population live in the urban areas. The rest reside basically in rural settings. The economy is based primarily on oil and agriculture, although the government receives enough revenue form oil. Nigeria, in comparison to the United States, can be classified as a traditional society with traditional norms. This is because Nigeria is still technologically underdeveloped and relatively unscientific. It is composed of members who are relatively more homogeneous in composition, but less cosmopolitan in comparison to the United States. The above traits imply that Nigeria, as a traditional system with emphasis on the traditional norms, will be less oriented to

Juicing For Your Soul

change. While a modern society, such as the United States, with modern norms, you will have the opposite characteristics. Norm is the established behavioral patterns for members of a given social system.

Nigerian economy is based upon oil, and Lagos—the former capital city—is as complex as New York City. Tall skyscrapers rise in a temperate climate similar to Los Angeles. Palm-lined drives wind around the city, past weathered brick buildings aged through Nigerian history. There have been may world influences in Nigeria. There still are. People travel from all over–Asia, Europe, and even North American–to settle and work in a city as beautiful and sophisticated as Lagos, Abuja, Jos Plateau, and some other parts of Nigerian cities. Lagos city was so congested that the government moved the capital to Abuja.

Due to the balmy weather, there is a tropical feel to Lagos, revealed in open-air markets which dot the thoroughfares of the city. The market offers native fare like the ugu, a relative to spinach. The seacoast offers up fresh pike, sea bass, and shell fish to be scrutinized by the fastidious family shopper. Hot peppers, mangoes, guava, pineapple, vegetables, tropical fruits, oranges, yams, and the unofficial national spice, curry, are bartered, bagged, and brought home for dinner.

The market is a colorful place where a little English mingles with dialect of Ibo, Yoruba, and Hausa. If you live long in Lagos, you will learn them all. And if you are like Phiner, and your parents are professionals, you will pick up other tongues in far-away places: Vietnamese, Korean, Russian, and French.

Biography

In the pristine city of Lagos in Nigeria there are many families; healthy, bright, happy people who live productively into their 100's. From this city has come one of the most delightful ladies anyone could ever have the pleasure to know...Phiner Dike (pronounced fena deekay). Her life has indeed been an odyssey.

Phiner is the oldest of seven children. She completed elementary and secondary school in Nigeria. During that time, Phiner was taught by her parents about the secrets of great nutrition, eating well, and refined culinary tastes.

Phiner now resides in the United States where she graduated from college with a degree in mass communication and public administration. Presently, she works as a model, actress, gourmet chef and Motivational Speaker. She has worked as a Broadcaster both on cable television, radio and has interviewed music and legendary Hollywood film stars such as Jane Powell, Michael McDonald (formerly of the Doobie Brothers), Marilyn McCoo and husband, Bill Davis, Jr., Red Buttons, Ann Jeffreys just to name a few. Sustained by an uplifting faith and disciplined approach to health, diet, art, self and society, Phiner's dedication to juicing is noticeable to close friends and family, for they all see her lifestyle revolve around her commitment to healthy living. Juicing has expounded her personal power with vibrant energy, happiness, and personal contentment.

Phiner's decision to grasp life and nurture herself appears to most as the road less traveled. Even though proper decisions to conglomerate her lifestyle have challenged her considerably, through dedication, commitment, and persistence, Phiner's aura radiates to

Juicing For Your Soul

everyone in her near proximity.

For years now, stemming from her prolific literary accounts of all she has learned and practiced regarding nutrition, Phiner has help people to assume a portion of responsibility for their own well-being. This philosophy was echoed in her radio and cable-TV broadcasts.

This 5 feet 5 inch tall, 100 pound Phiner now offers a book that combines her proven expertise in cooking and beauty. *Juicing For Your Soul: An Invitation to Health and Longevity* draws from both segments of Phiner's life – the old wisdom of her childhood in Lagos, and from her cosmopolitan life in America. Anyone savvy enough to read this and other books by Phiner Dike and follow the sensible, simple regimes by which she lives can also enjoy the health and vitality of such an incredible lady.

We, as a nation of "instant" everything, or as health conscious individuals, cannot afford to ignore this wealth of guidance to a fuller, better life.

Biography by
Judith Drake, Author

Juicing For Your Soul

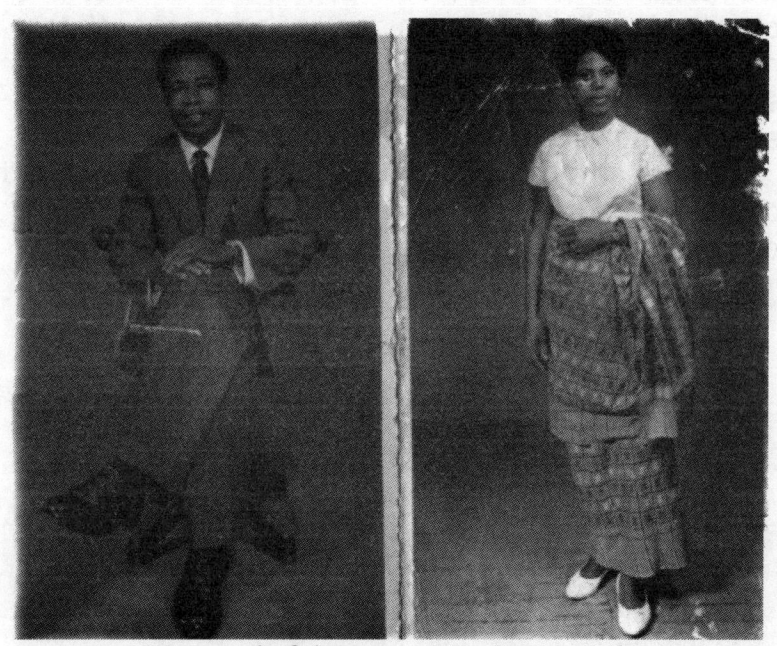

My wonderful parents: Mr. & Mrs. Dike

Juicing For Your Soul

Calorie Count Section

Serv. Size: 1 lg. Apple,

Calories: 81.4, Carbohydrates (gm) 21, Protein (gm) 0.3, Total Fat (gm), 0.5, Saturated Fat (gm), 0.1, Cholesterol (mg) 0, Sodium (mg) 0, Potassium (mg) 158.7, Iron (mg) 0.2, Dietary Fiber (gm), 3.7.

Serving Size: 1 cup Alpha sprouts,

Calories: 4.9, Carbohydrates (gm) 0.6, Protein (gm) 0.7, Total Fat (gm), 0.1, Saturated Fat (gm), 0, Cholesterol (mg) 0, Sodium (mg) 1, Potassium (mg) 13.4, Iron (mg) 0.2, Dietary Fiber (gm), 0.4.

Serving Size: Apricot,

Calories: 16.8, Carbohydrates (gm) 3.9, Protein (gm) 0.5, Total Fat (gm), 0.1, Saturated Fat (gm), 0, Cholesterol (mg) 0, Sodium (mg) 0.4, Potassium (mg) 103.6, Iron (mg) 0.2, Dietary Fiber (gm), 0.8.

Serving Size: 1 lb. Asparagus,

Calories: 2.1, Carbohydrates (gm) 0.4, Protein (gm) 0.2, Total Fat (gm), 0, Saturated Fat (gm), 0, Cholesterol (mg) 0, Sodium (mg) 0.2, Potassium (mg) 24.6, Iron (mg) 0.1, Dietary Fiber (gm), 0.2.

Serving Size: 1 oz. Basil

Calories: 6, Carbohydrates (gm) 1.1, Protein (gm) 4, Total Fat (gm), 0.1, Saturated Fat (gm), 0, Cholesterol (mg) 0, Sodium (mg) 0, Potassium (mg) 62, Iron (mg) 2.2, Dietary Fiber (gm), 0.

Serving Size: 1 med. Beet (100g)

Calories: 50, Carbohydrates (gm) 21, Protein (gm) 0.3, Total Fat (gm), 0.5, Saturated Fat (gm), 0, Cholesterol (mg) 0, Sodium (mg) 0, Potassium (mg) 0, Iron (mg) 0, Dietary Fiber (gm), 0.

Serving Size: 1 cup Blackberries,

Calories: 37.4, Carbohydrates (gm) 9.2, Protein (gm) 0.5, Total Fat (gm), 0.3, Saturated Fat (gm), 0, Cholesterol (mg) 0, Sodium (mg) 0, Potassium (mg) 141.1, Iron (mg) 0.4, Dietary Fiber (gm), 3.8

Serving Size:1 lb. Broccoli,
Calories: 12.3, Carbohydrates (gm) 2.3, Protein (gm) 1.3, Total Fat (gm), 0.2, Saturated Fat (gm), 0, Cholesterol (mg) 0, Sodium (mg)11.9, Potassium (mg) 143, Iron (mg) 0.4, Dietary Fiber (gm), 1.3.

Serving Size: 1 med. Cantaloupe,

Calories: 29.7, Carbohydrates (gm) 7.1, Protein (gm) 0.7, Total Fat (gm), 0.2, Saturated Fat (gm), 0.1, Cholesterol (mg) 0, Sodium (mg) 7.7, Potassium (mg) 262.7, Iron (mg) 0.2, Dietary Fiber (gm), 0.7.

Serving Size: 2 med. Carrots

Calories: 110.4, Carbohydrates (gm) 8.2, Protein (gm) 0.6, Total Fat (gm), 6.7, Saturated

Juicing For Your Soul

Fat (gm), 1.1, Cholesterol (mg) 0, Sodium (mg) 46.1, Potassium (mg) 179.6, Iron (mg) 0.3, Dietary Fiber (gm), 2.2..

Serving Size: 1 cup Cherries,

Calories: 42.5, Carbohydrates (gm) 9.8, Protein (gm) 0.7, Total Fat (gm), 0.6, Saturated Fat (gm), 0.1, Cholesterol (mg) 0, Sodium (mg) 0, Potassium (mg) 132.2, Iron (mg) 0.2, Dietary Fiber (gm), 1.4.

Serving Size: 1 cup Chives,

Calories: 0.9, Carbohydrates (gm) 0.1, Protein (gm) 0.1, Total Fat (gm), 0, Saturated Fat (gm), 0, Cholesterol (mg) 0.1, Sodium (mg) 0, Potassium (mg) 8.9, Iron (mg) 0, Dietary Fiber (gm), 0.

Serving Size: 1 cup Cilantro,

Calories: 2.2, Carbohydrates (gm) 0.4, Protein (gm) 0.2, Total Fat (gm), 0.2, Saturated Fat (gm), 0, Cholesterol (mg) 0, Sodium (mg) 0, Potassium (mg) 45.9, Iron (mg) 0.2, Dietary Fiber (gm), 0.3

Serving Size: ½ lb. Collards,

Calories: 5.4, Carbohydrates (gm) 1, Protein (gm) 0.4, Total Fat (gm), 0.1, Saturated Fat (gm), 0, Cholesterol (mg) 0, Sodium (mg) 3.6, Potassium (mg) 30.4, Iron (mg) 0, Dietary Fiber (gm), 0.6

Serving Size: 1 cup Cranberries,

Calories: 4.4, Carbohydrates (gm) 1.1, Protein (gm) -, Total Fat (gm) 0, Saturated Fat (gm), 0, Cholesterol (mg) -, Sodium (mg) 0.1, Potassium (mg) 6.4, Iron (mg) 0, Dietary Fiber (gm), 0.4.

Serving Size: 1 lg. Cucumbers,

Calories: 7.2, Carbohydrates (gm) 1.5, Protein (gm) 0.3, Total Fat (gm), 0.1, Saturated Fat (gm), 0, Cholesterol (mg) 0, Sodium (mg) 1.2, Potassium (mg) 88.8, Iron (mg) 0.1, Dietary Fiber (gm),0.

Serving Size: ½ lb. Dandelion greens,

Calories: 12.6, Carbohydrates (gm) 2.6, Protein (gm) 0.8, Total Fat (gm), 0.2, Saturated Fat (gm), 0.2 Cholesterol (mg) 0, Sodium (mg) 21.3, Potassium (mg) 111.2, Iron (mg) 0.9 Dietary Fiber (gm), 1..

Serving Size: ½ lb. Endive,

Calories: 7.2, Carbohydrates (gm) 1.4, Protein (gm) 0.6, Total Fat (gm), 0.1, Saturated Fat (gm), 0, Cholesterol (mg) 0, Sodium (mg) 0, Potassium (mg) 10, Iron (mg) 0136.5, Dietary Fiber (gm), 0.4.

Serving Size: 6 cloves Garlic,

Calories: 4.5, Carbohydrates (gm) 1, Protein (gm) 0.2, Total Fat (gm), 0, Saturated Fat (gm), 0, Cholesterol (mg) 0, Sodium (mg) 0.5, Potassium (mg) 12, Iron (mg) 0.1, Dietary Fiber (gm), 0.1.

Juicing For Your Soul

Serving Size: 3 lg. Grapefruit,

Calories: 41, Carbohydrates (gm) 10.3, Protein (gm) 0.8, Total Fat (gm), 0.1, Saturated Fat (gm), 0, Cholesterol (mg) 0, Sodium (mg) 0, Potassium (mg) 177.9, Iron (mg) 0.1, Dietary Fiber (gm), 1.4

Serving Size: 1 cup Grapes,

Calories: 56.8, Carbohydrates (gm) 14.2, Protein (gm) 0.5, Total Fat (gm), 0.5, Saturated Fat (gm), 0.2, Cholesterol (mg) 0, Sodium (mg) 1.6, Potassium (mg) 148, Iron (mg) 0.2, Dietary Fiber (gm), 0.8

Serving Size: ½ lb. Jicama,

Calories: 24.7, Carbohydrates (gm) 5.7, Protein (gm) 0.5, Total Fat (gm), 0.1, Saturated Fat (gm), 0, Cholesterol (mg) 0, Sodium (mg) 2.6, Potassium (mg) 97.5, Iron (mg) 0.4, Dietary Fiber (gm), 3.2

Serving Size: 3 Kiwi fruit,

Calories: 46.4, Carbohydrates (gm) 11.3, Protein (gm) 0.8, Total Fat (gm), 0.3, Saturated Fat (gm), 0, Cholesterol (mg) 0, Sodium (mg) 3.8, Potassium (mg) 252.3, Iron (mg) 0.3, Dietary Fiber (gm), 2.6

Serving Size: ½ lb. Kohlrabi,

Calories: 18.4, Carbohydrates (gm) 4.2, Protein (gm) 1.2, Total Fat (gm), 0.1, Saturated Fat (gm), 0, Cholesterol (mg) 0, Sodium (mg) 13.6, Potassium (mg) 238, Iron (mg)

0.3, Dietary Fiber (gm), 2.4

Serving Size: Leek,

Calories: 5.5, Carbohydrates (gm) 1.3, Protein (gm) 0.1, Total Fat (gm), 0, Saturated Fat (gm), 0, Cholesterol (mg) 0, Sodium (mg) 1.8, Potassium (mg) 16.2, Iron (mg) 0.2, Dietary Fiber (gm), 0.2

Serving Size: 1 whole Lemon,

Calories: 2, Carbohydrates (gm) 0.7, Protein (gm) 0.1, Total Fat (gm), 0, Saturated Fat (gm), 0, Cholesterol (mg) 0, Sodium (mg) 0.1, Potassium (mg) 9.7, Iron (mg) 0, Dietary Fiber (gm), 0.2.

Serving Size: ½ lb. Lettuce, arugula,

Calories: 2.3, Carbohydrates (gm) 0.3, Protein (gm) 0.2, Total Fat (gm), 0.1, Saturated Fat (gm), 0, Cholesterol (mg) 0, Sodium (mg) 2.4, Potassium (mg) 33.2, Iron (mg) 0.1, Dietary Fiber (gm), 0.1

Serving Size: ½ lb. Lettuce, Boston,

Calories: 7.2, Carbohydrates (gm) 1.3, Protein (gm) 0.7, Total Fat (gm), 0.1, Saturated Fat (gm), 0, Cholesterol (mg) 0, Sodium (mg) 2.8, Potassium (mg) 141.4, Iron (mg) 0.2, Dietary Fiber (gm), 0.6

Serving Size: 1 Lime,

Calories: 2.4, Carbohydrates (gm) 0.8, Protein (gm) 0.1, Total Fat (gm), 0, Saturated Fat (gm), 0, Cholesterol (mg)

0, Sodium (mg) 0.2, Potassium (mg) 8.2, Iron (mg) 0, Dietary Fiber (gm), 0.2.

Serving Size: Mango,

Calories: 67, Carbohydrates (gm) 17.5, Protein (gm) 0.5, Total Fat (gm), 0.3, Saturated Fat (gm), 0.1, Cholesterol (mg) 0, Sodium (mg) 2.1, Potassium (mg) 160.7, Iron (mg) 0.1, Dietary Fiber (gm), 1.9.

Serving Size: 1 oz. Marjoram

Calories: 2, Carbohydrates (gm) 1.1, Protein (gm) 2.5, Total Fat (gm), 0, Saturated Fat (gm), 0, Cholesterol (mg) 0, Sodium (mg) 0, Potassium (mg) 9, Iron (mg) 20, Dietary Fiber (gm), 23.

Serving Size: Mustard greens,

Calories: 67, Carbohydrates (gm) 17.5, Protein (gm) 0.8, Total Fat (gm), 0.1, Saturated Fat (gm), 0, Cholesterol (mg) 0, Sodium (mg) 7, Potassium (mg) 99.1, Iron (mg) 0.4, Dietary Fiber (gm), 0.9

Serving Size: Nectarine,

Calories: 66.6, Carbohydrates (gm) 16, Protein (gm) 1.3, Total Fat (gm), 0.6, Saturated Fat (gm), 0.1, Cholesterol (mg) 0, Sodium (mg) 5.7, Potassium (mg) 0, Iron (mg) 0.2, Dietary Fiber (gm), 2.2

Serving Size: 1 Red Onion,

Calories: 5.3, Carbohydrates (gm) 1.2, Protein (gm) 0.2,

Total Fat (gm), 0, Saturated Fat (gm), 0, Cholesterol (mg) 0, Sodium (mg) 0.4, Potassium (mg) 22, Iron (mg) 0, Dietary Fiber (gm) 0.

Serving Size: 1 bunch Onions, (aka scallions),

Calories: 4.8, Carbohydrates (gm) 1.1, Protein (gm) 0.3, Total Fat (gm), 0, Saturated Fat (gm), 0, Cholesterol (mg) 0, Sodium (mg) 2.4, Potassium (mg) 41.4, Iron (mg) 0.2, Dietary Fiber (gm), 0.4

Serving Size: 3 lg. Oranges,

Calories: 61.6, Carbohydrates (gm) 15.4, Protein (gm) 1.2, Total Fat (gm), 0.2, Saturated Fat (gm), 0, Cholesterol (mg) 0, Sodium (mg) 0, Potassium (mg) 237.1, Iron (mg) 0.1, Dietary Fiber (gm), 3.1.

Serving Size: 1 cup Parsley

Calories: 1.4, Carbohydrates (gm) 0.3, Protein (gm) 0.1, Total Fat (gm), 0, Saturated Fat (gm), 0, Cholesterol (mg) 0, Sodium (mg) 2.2, Potassium (mg) 22.2, Iron (mg) 0.2, Dietary Fiber (gm), 0.1

Serving Size: 4 Peaches

Calories: 42.1, Carbohydrates (gm) 10.9, Protein (gm) 0.7, Total Fat (gm), 0.1, Saturated Fat (gm), 0, Cholesterol (mg) 0, Sodium (mg) 0, Potassium (mg) 193.1, Iron (mg) 0.1, Dietary Fiber (gm), 2.

Juicing For Your Soul

Serving Size: Pear, Japanese,

Calories: 3.8, Carbohydrates (gm) 1, Protein (gm) 0, Total Fat (gm), 0, Saturated Fat (gm), 0, Cholesterol (mg) 0, Sodium (mg) 2.6, Potassium (mg) 10.9, Iron (mg) 0.3, Dietary Fiber (gm), 0.3

Serving Size: Peas, green,

Calories: 58.3, Carbohydrates (gm) 10.4, Protein (gm) 3.9, Total Fat (gm), 0.3, Saturated Fat (gm), 0.1, Cholesterol (mg) 0, Sodium (mg) 3.6, Potassium (mg) 175.7, Iron (mg) 1.1, Dietary Fiber (gm), 3.7

Serving Size: 5 lg. Peppers, sweet, green,

Calories: 20.3, Carbohydrates (gm) 4.8, Protein (gm) 0.7, Total Fat (gm), 0.1, Saturated Fat (gm), 0, Cholesterol (mg) 0, Sodium (mg) 1.5, Potassium (mg) 132.8, Iron (mg) 0.3, Dietary Fiber (gm), 1.4

Serving Size: Pineapple, (3 slices)

Calories: 38.2, Carbohydrates (gm) 9.7, Protein (gm) 0.3, Total Fat (gm), 0.3, Saturated Fat (gm) 0, Cholesterol (mg) 0, Sodium (mg) 0.8, Potassium (mg) 88.1, Iron (mg) 0.3, Dietary Fiber (gm), 0.9.

Serving Size: 1 cup Raspberries, black,

Calories: 32.8, Carbohydrates (gm) 7.8, Protein (gm) 0.6, Total Fat (gm), 0.4, Saturated Fat (gm), 0, Cholesterol (mg) 0, Sodium (mg) 0, Potassium (mg) 101.8, Iron (mg) 0.4, Dietary Fiber (gm), 4.6

Serving Size: 1 cup Radish,

Calories: 11.6, Carbohydrates (gm) 2.1, Protein (gm) 0.3, Total Fat (gm), 0.3, Saturated Fat (gm), 0, Cholesterol (mg) 0, Sodium (mg) 13.9, Potassium (mg) 134.6, Iron (mg) 0.2, Dietary Fiber (gm), 0.9.

Serving Size: 2 lg. Rhubarb,

Calories: 10.7, Carbohydrates (gm) 2.3, Protein (gm) 0.5, Total Fat (gm), 0.1, Saturated Fat (gm), 0, Cholesterol (mg) 2, Sodium (mg) 5.7, Potassium (mg) 146.9, Iron (mg) 0.1, Dietary Fiber (gm), 0.9

Serving Size: 2 lg. Rutabaga,

Calories: 25.2, Carbohydrates (gm) 5.7, Protein (gm) 0.8, Total Fat (gm), 0.1, Saturated Fat (gm), 0, Cholesterol (mg) 0, Sodium (mg) 14, Potassium (mg) 235.9, Iron (mg) 0.4, Dietary Fiber (gm), 1.8

Serving Size: Rosemary, 1oz.

Calories: 12, Carbohydrates (gm) 21, Protein (gm) 0.3, Total Fat (gm), 0, Saturated Fat (gm), 0, Cholesterol (mg) 0, Sodium (mg) 0, Potassium (mg) 0, Iron (mg) 0, Dietary Fiber (gm), 0.

Serving Size: Snowpeas, (pead pod),

Calories: 13.4, Carbohydrates (gm) 2.4, Protein (gm) 0.9, Total Fat (gm), 0, Saturated Fat (gm), 0, Cholesterol (mg) 0, Sodium (mg) 1.3, Potassium (mg) 64, Iron (mg) 0.7, Dietary Fiber (gm), 0.8

Juicing For Your Soul

Serving Size: 1 lb. Spinach,

Calories: 6.6, Carbohydrates (gm) 1.1, Protein (gm) 0.9, Total Fat (gm), 0.1, Saturated Fat (gm), 0, Cholesterol (mg) 0, Sodium (mg) 23.7, Potassium (mg) 167.4, Iron (mg) 0.8, Dietary Fiber (gm), 0.8

Serving Size: Stberries,

Calories: 21.6, Carbohydrates (gm) 5.1, Protein (gm) 0.4, Total Fat (gm), 0.3, Saturated Fat (gm), 0, Cholesterol (mg) 0, Sodium (mg) 0.7, Potassium (mg)119.5, Iron (mg) 0.3, Dietary Fiber (gm), 1.7

Serving Size: 10 small Tangerine,

Calories: 37, Carbohydrates (gm) 9.4, Protein (gm) 0.5, Total Fat (gm), 0.2, Saturated Fat (gm), 0, Cholesterol (mg) 0, Sodium (mg) 0.8, Potassium (mg) 131.9, Iron (mg) 0.1, Dietary Fiber (gm), 1.9

Serving Size: 4 lg. Tomatoes,

Calories: 25.8, Carbohydrates (gm) 5.7, Protein (gm) 1, Total Fat (gm), 0.4, Saturated Fat (gm), 0.4 Cholesterol (mg) 0.1, Sodium (mg) 11.1, Potassium (mg) 273.1, Iron (mg) 0.6, Dietary Fiber (gm), 1.4

Serving Size: 1 lb. Turnip,

Calories: 17.6, Carbohydrates (gm) 4, Protein (gm) 0.6, Total Fat (gm), 0.1, Saturated Fat (gm), 0, Cholesterol (mg) 0, Sodium (mg) 43.6, Potassium (mg) 124.2, Iron (mg) 0.2, Dietary Fiber (gm), 1.2

Serving Size: Watercress,

Calories: 1.9, Carbohydrates (gm) 0.2, Protein (gm) 0.4, Total Fat (gm), 0, Saturated Fat (gm), 0, Cholesterol (mg) 0, Sodium (mg) 7, Potassium (mg) 56.1, Iron (mg) 0, Dietary Fiber (gm).

Serving Size: Watermelon (286 gm), (3 slices)

Calories: 91.5, Carbohydrates (gm) 20.5, Protein (gm) 1.8, Total Fat (gm), 1.2, Saturated Fat (gm), 0.1, Cholesterol (mg) 0, Sodium (mg) 5.7, Potassium (mg) 331.8, Iron (mg) 0.5, Dietary Fiber (gm), 1.4.

Serving Size: 3 lg. red-skinned potato, any color but white with or without peel (assume peel not eaten).

Calories: 96.4, Carbohydrates (gm) 21.9, Protein (gm) 2.5, Total Fat (gm), 0.1, Saturated Fat (gm), 0, Cholesterol (mg) 0, Sodium (mg) 7.3, Potassium (mg) 662.5, Iron (mg) 0.9, Dietary Fiber (gm), 0.

Juicing For Your Soul

Notes

Notes

Juicing For Your Soul

Notes

Notes